Daily Gratitude Journal

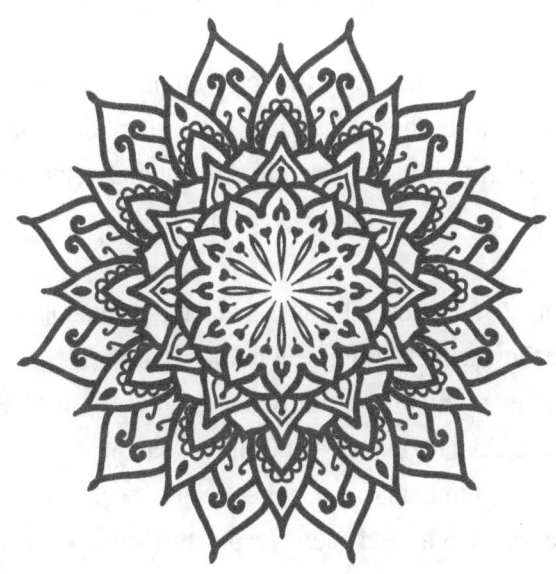

Thank You!

© Copyright 2021 - All rights reserved.

You may not reproduce, duplicate or send the contents of this book without direct written permission from the author. You cannot hereby despite any circumstance blame the publisher or hold him or her to legal responsibility for any reparation, compensations, or monetary forfeiture owing to the information included herein, either in a direct or an indirect way.

Legal Notice: This book has copyright protection. You can use the book for personal purpose. You should not sell, use, alter, distribute, quote, take excerpts or paraphrase in part or whole the material contained in this book without obtaining the permission of the author first.

Disclaimer Notice: You must take note that the information in this document is for casual reading and entertainment purposes only.
We have made every attempt to provide accurate, up to date and reliable information. We do not express or imply guarantees of any kind. The persons who read admit that the writer is not occupied in giving legal, financial, medical or other advice. We put this book content by sourcing various places.

Please consult a licensed professional before you try any techniques shown in this book. By going through this document, the book lover comes to an agreement that under no situation is the author accountable for any forfeiture, direct or indirect, which they may incur because of the use of material contained in this document, including, but not limited to, — errors, omissions, or inaccuracies.

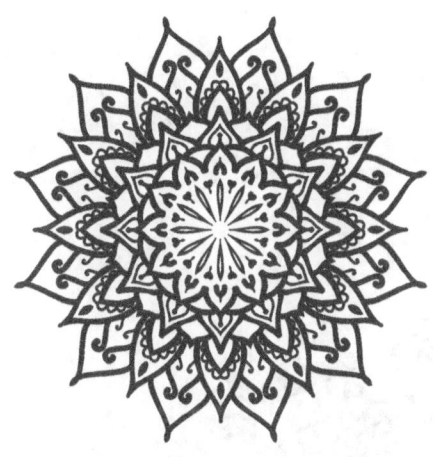

This Gratitude Journal Belongs To

....

....

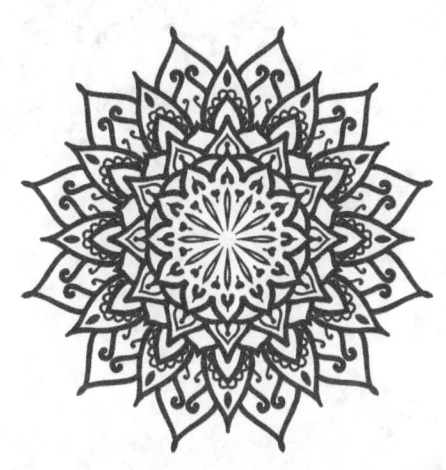

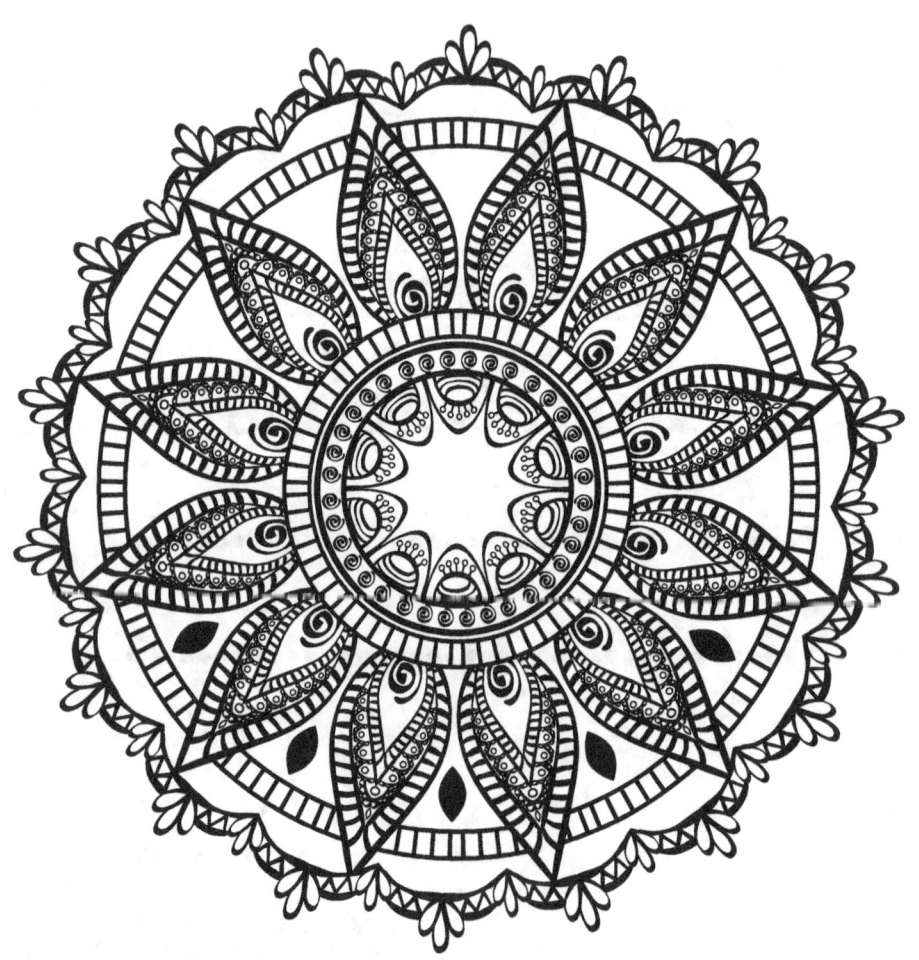

"Be thankful for what you have; you'll end up having more. ,If you concentrate on what you don't have, you will never, ever have enough."
Oprah Winfrey

"As we express our gratitude, we must never forget that the highest appreciation is not to utter words but to live by them."
John F. Kennedy

"Start each day with a positive thought and a grateful heart."
Roy T. Bennett

Be Grateful!!!

"Thankfulness is the beginning of gratitude. Gratitude is the completion of thankfulness. Thankfulness may consist merely of words. Gratitude is shown in acts." Henri Frederic Amiel

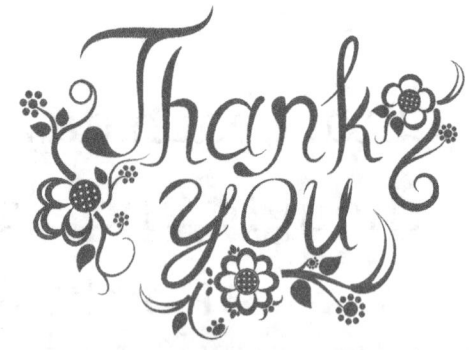

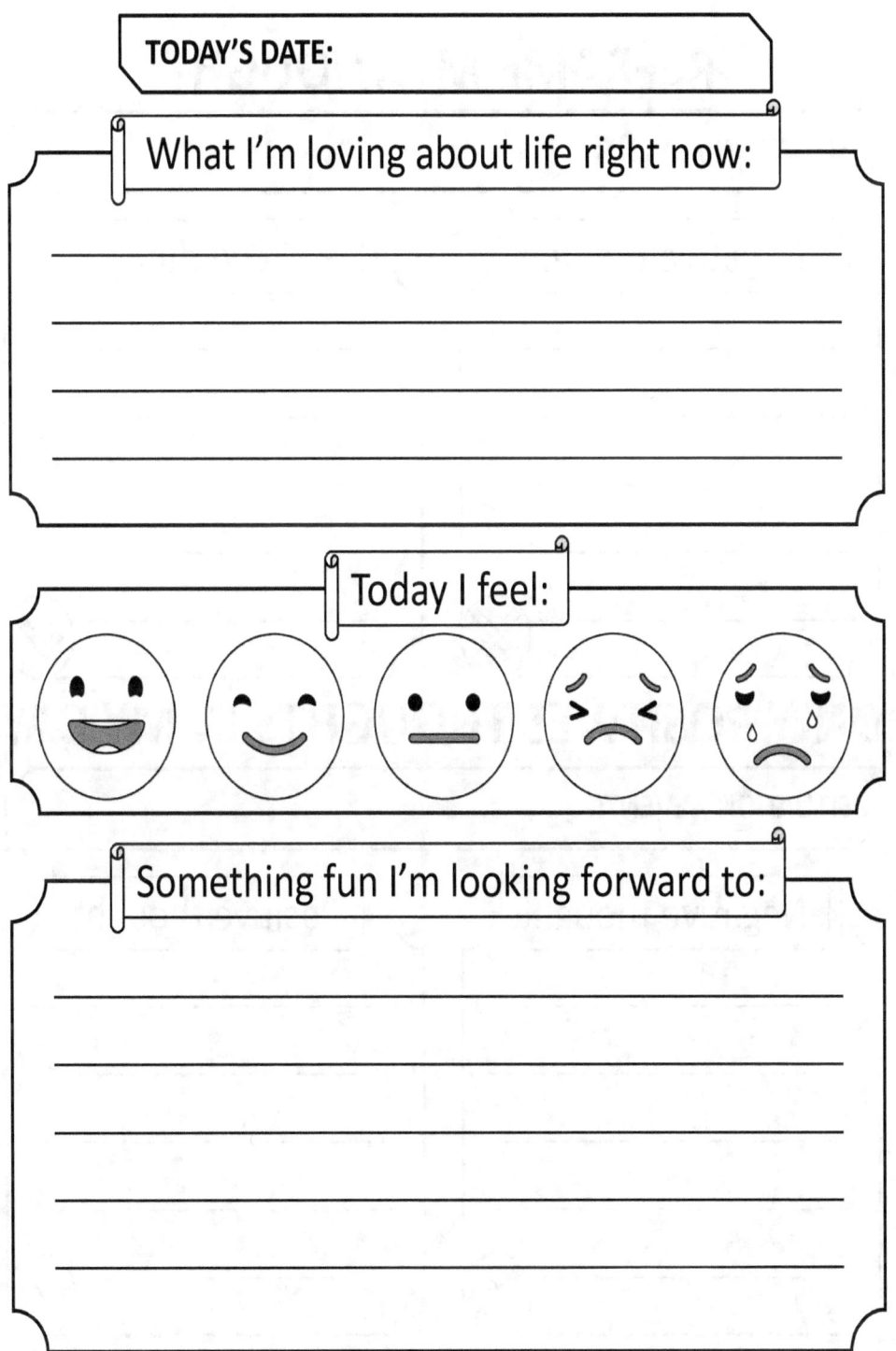

REFRAME MY THOUGHT

SITUATION / EVENT:

Negative thought
_____
_____
_____
_____
_____
❌

Positive thought
_____
_____
_____
_____
_____
✓

ONLY POSITIVES THOUGHTS IN MY DAY

SITUATION / EVENT:

Negative thought
_____
_____
_____
_____
_____
❌

Positive thought
_____
_____
_____
_____
_____
✓

TODAY'S DATE:

When I'm tired, I: _____
_____
_____

When I'm stressed, I: _____
_____
_____

When I'm upset, I: _____
_____
_____

When I'm angry, I: _____
_____
_____

When I feel down, I: _____
_____
_____

MY CONFIDENCE GOALS

What I want to achieve: _____

By: _____

Challenges: _____
_____

What I need to do:

_____
_____
_____
_____
_____
_____
_____

Result: _____
_____

Key takeaway: _____
_____

TODAY'S DATE:

What I want to achieve: _____

By: _____

Challenges: _____

_____

What I need to do:

_____
_____
_____
_____
_____
_____
_____
_____

Result: _____

_____

Key takeaway: _____

_____

I'M GRATEFUL

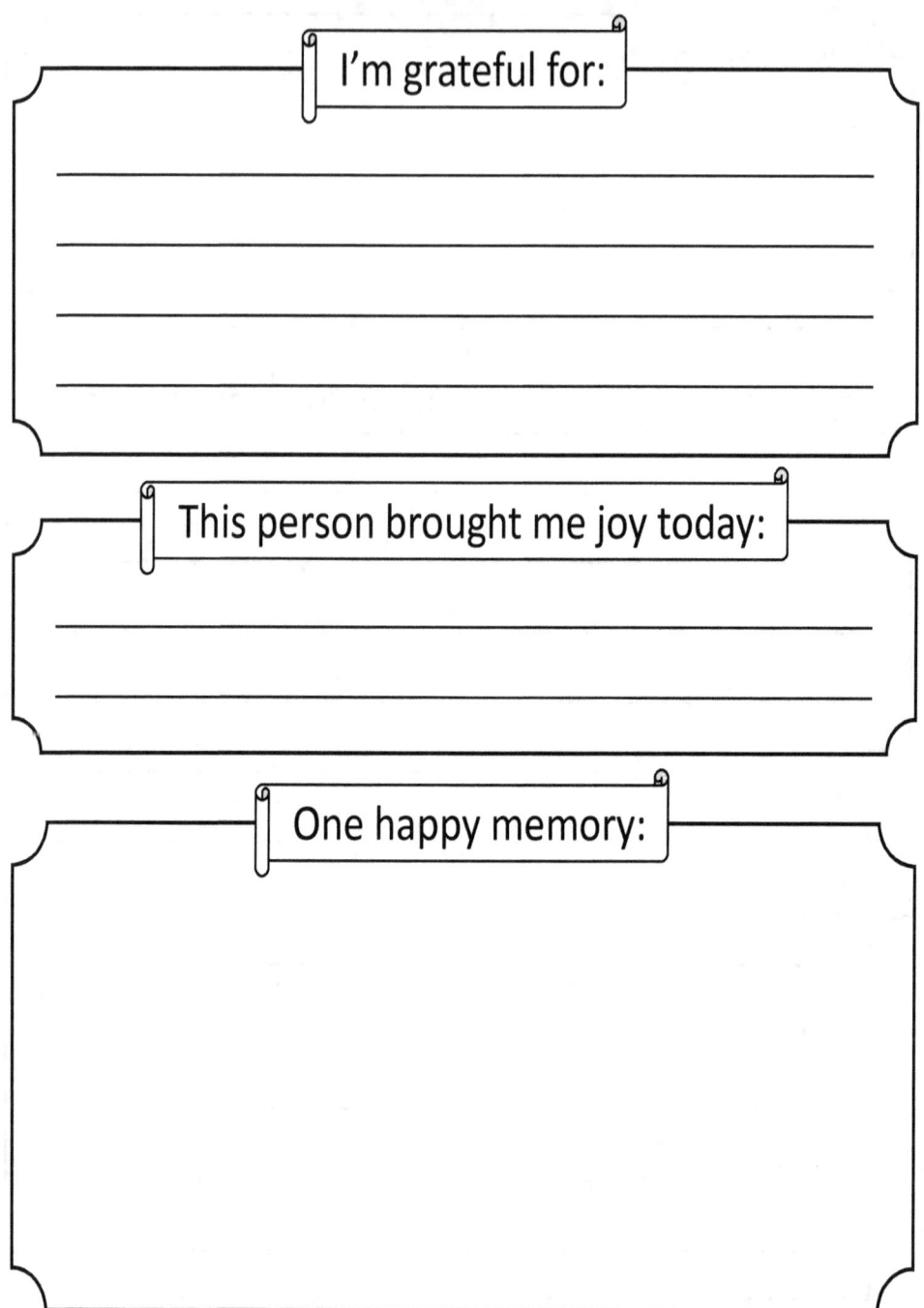

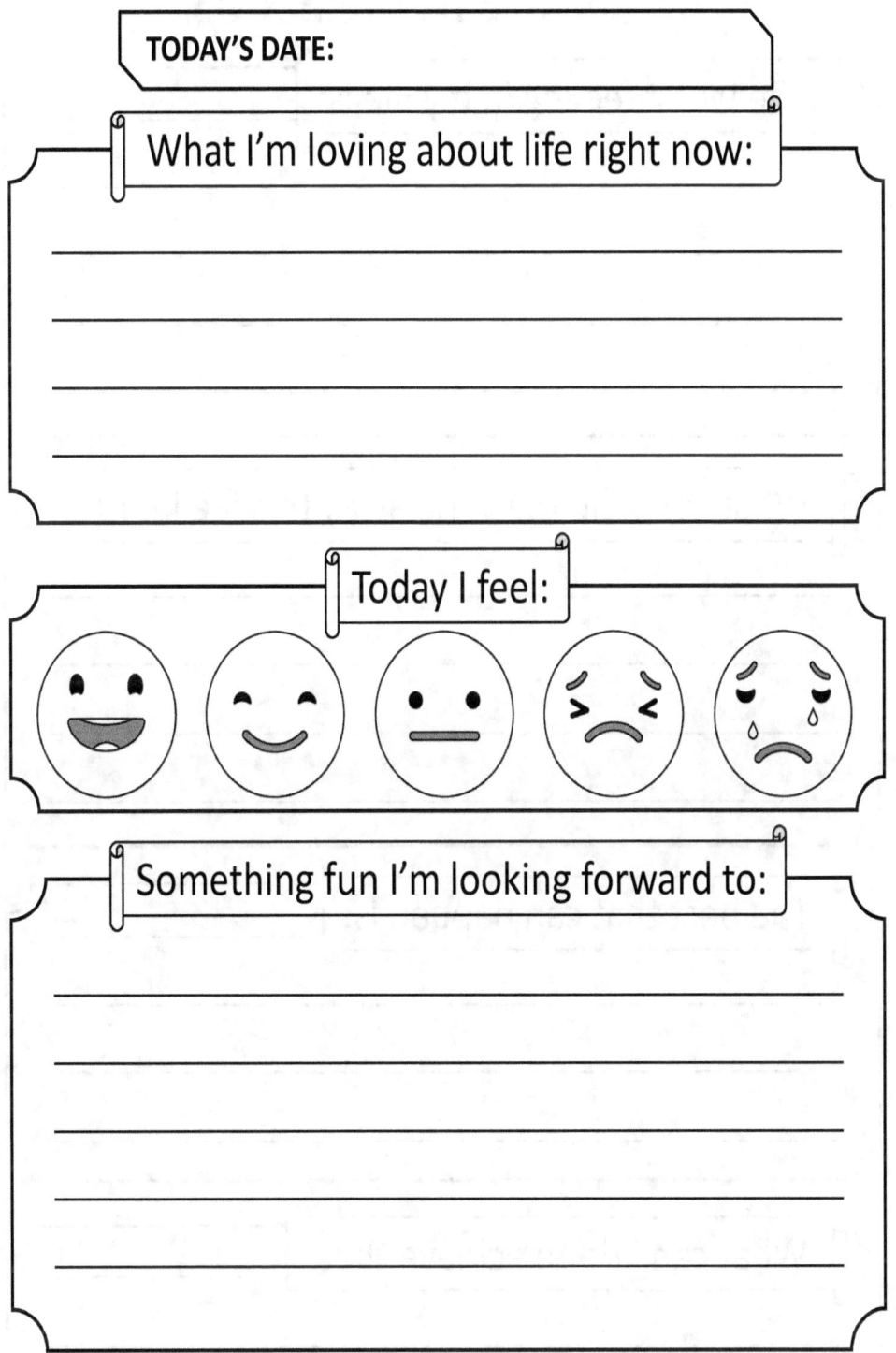

MANAGE MY FEELING

The worst feeling in my life is:

What can help me wipe away this feeling:

The best that can happen is:

What can I do to achieve that:

TODAY'S DATE:

The best feeling in my life is:

___

Say something nice about you/your life:

I'M GRATEFUL

I'm grateful for:

_____

_____

_____

_____

This person brought me joy today:

_____

_____

One happy memory:

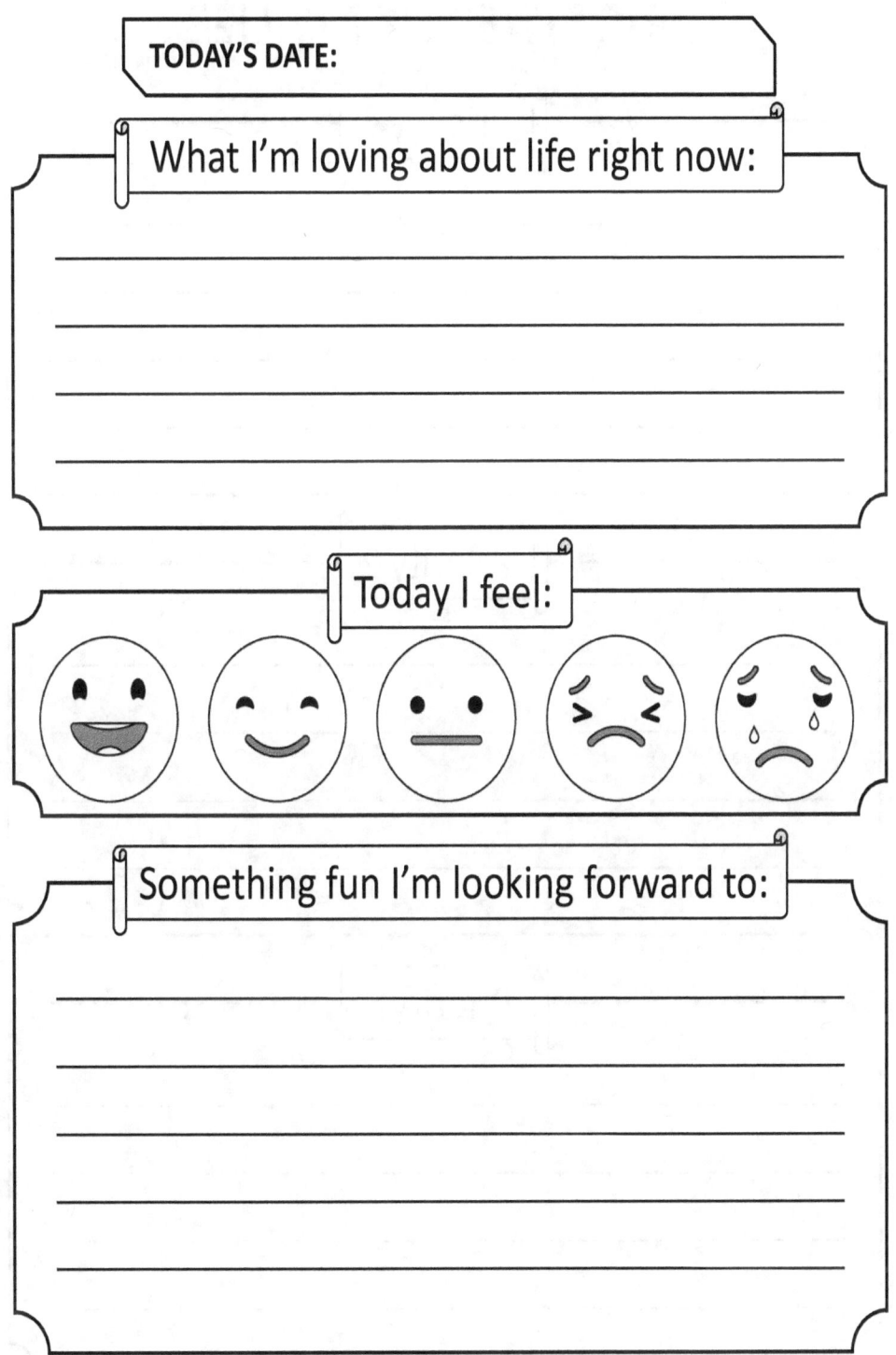

PRIORITIES OF MY LIFE

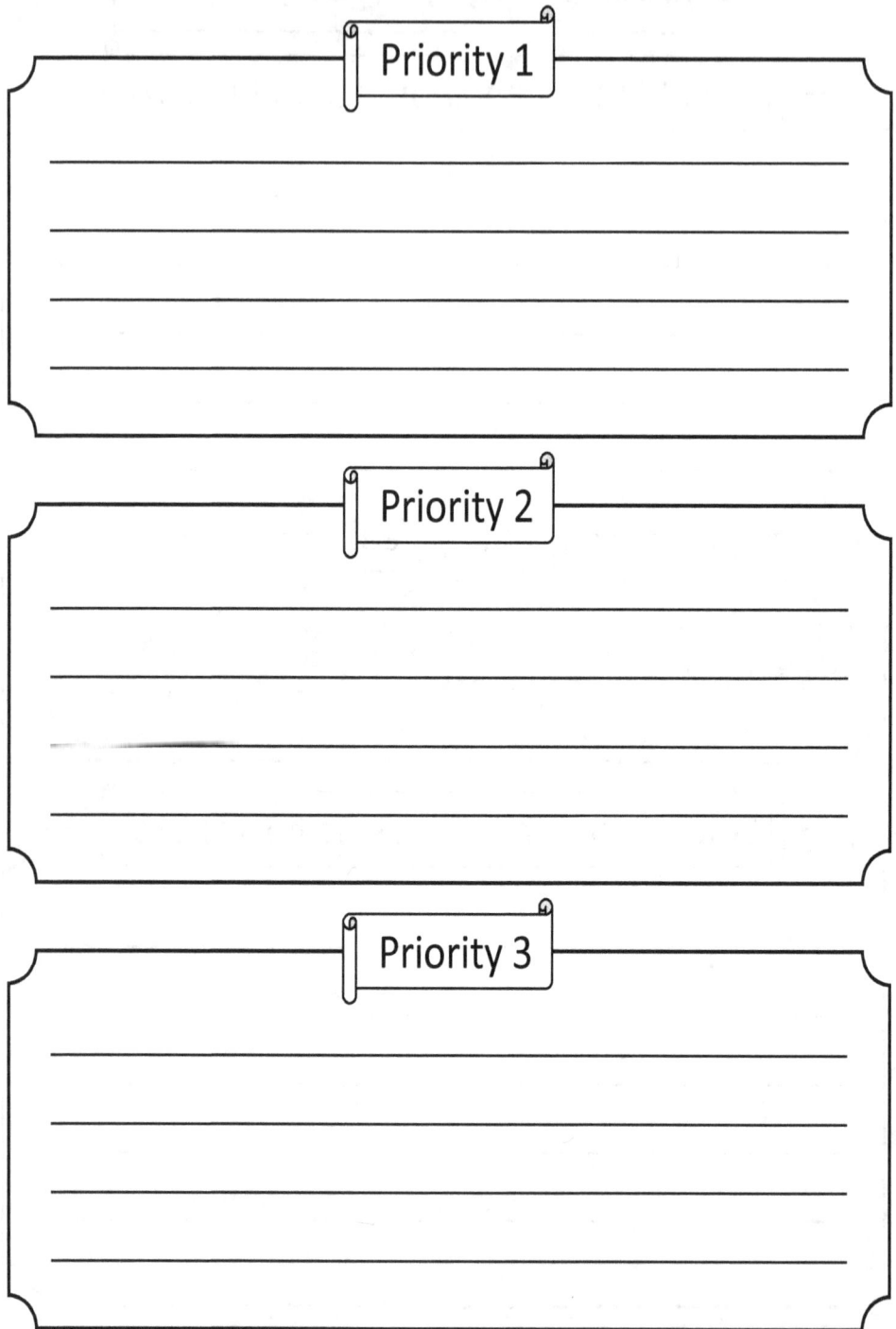

TODAY'S DATE:

Priority 4

_____
_____
_____
_____

Priority 5

_____
_____
_____
_____

Priority 6

_____
_____
_____
_____

SHARE MORE ABOUT YOUR SELF

I'm someone who loves:

_____
_____
_____
_____

I'm someone who can:

_____
_____
_____
_____

I'm someone who has:

_____
_____
_____
_____

TODAY'S DATE:

I'm someone who wishes:

I'm someone who is thankful for:

I'm someone who never forgets to:

I'M GRATEFUL

I'm grateful for:

_____

_____

_____

_____

This person brought me joy today:

_____

_____

One happy memory:

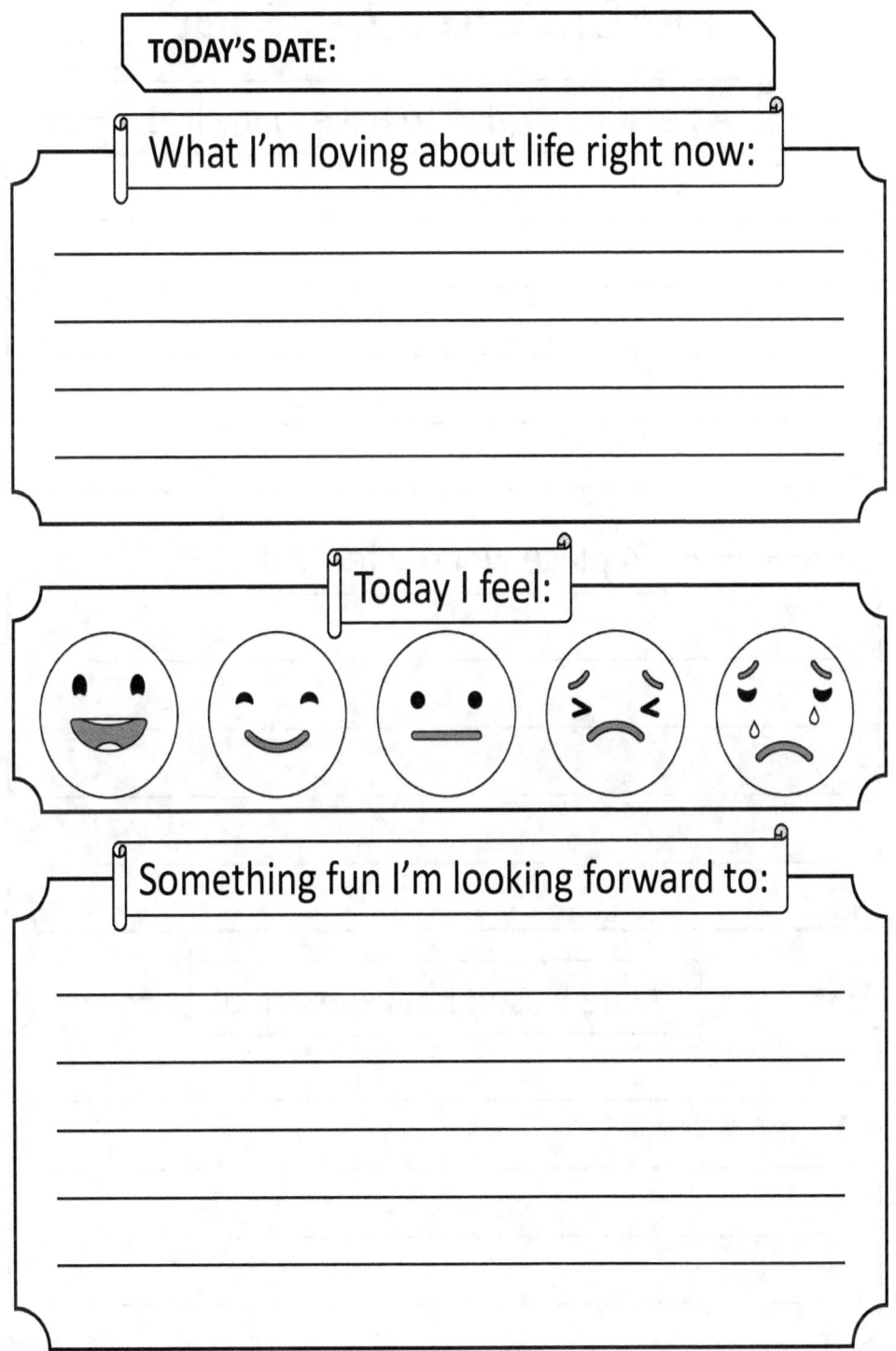

PRACTICING GRATITUDE

A person I'm glad to have in my live:

_____
_____
_____
_____

A place where I feel safe:

_____
_____
_____
_____

A life lesson I have learned:

_____
_____
_____
_____

TODAY'S DATE:

A characteristic of my home that I love:

_____
_____
_____
_____

My favorite aspect of my personality:

_____
_____
_____
_____

A book that I loved reading:

_____
_____
_____
_____

PRACTICING GRATITUDE

My favorite song that improves my mind:

_____
_____
_____
_____

A memory that makes me smile:

_____
_____
_____
_____

My favorite food or meal:

_____
_____
_____
_____

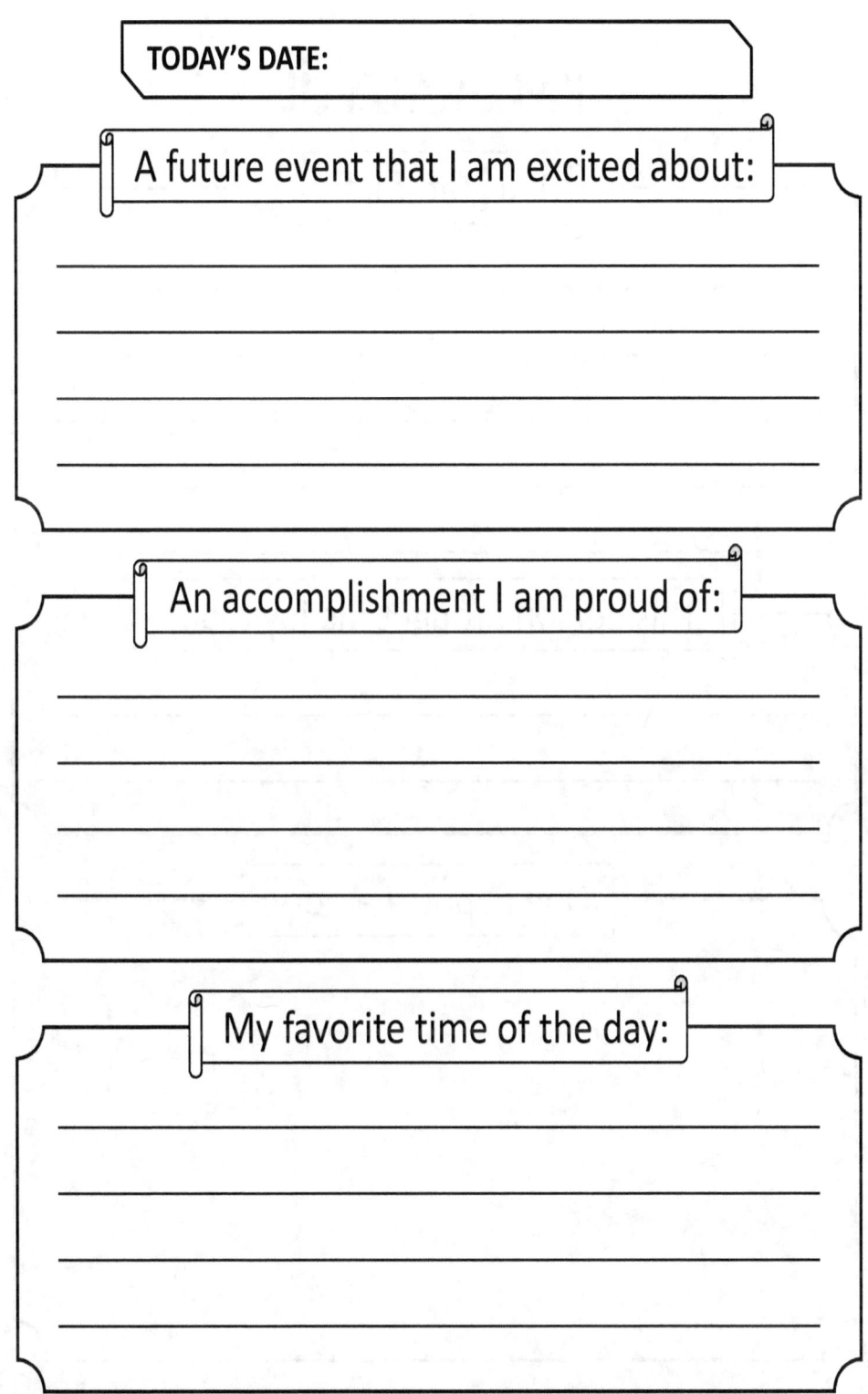

I'M GRATEFUL

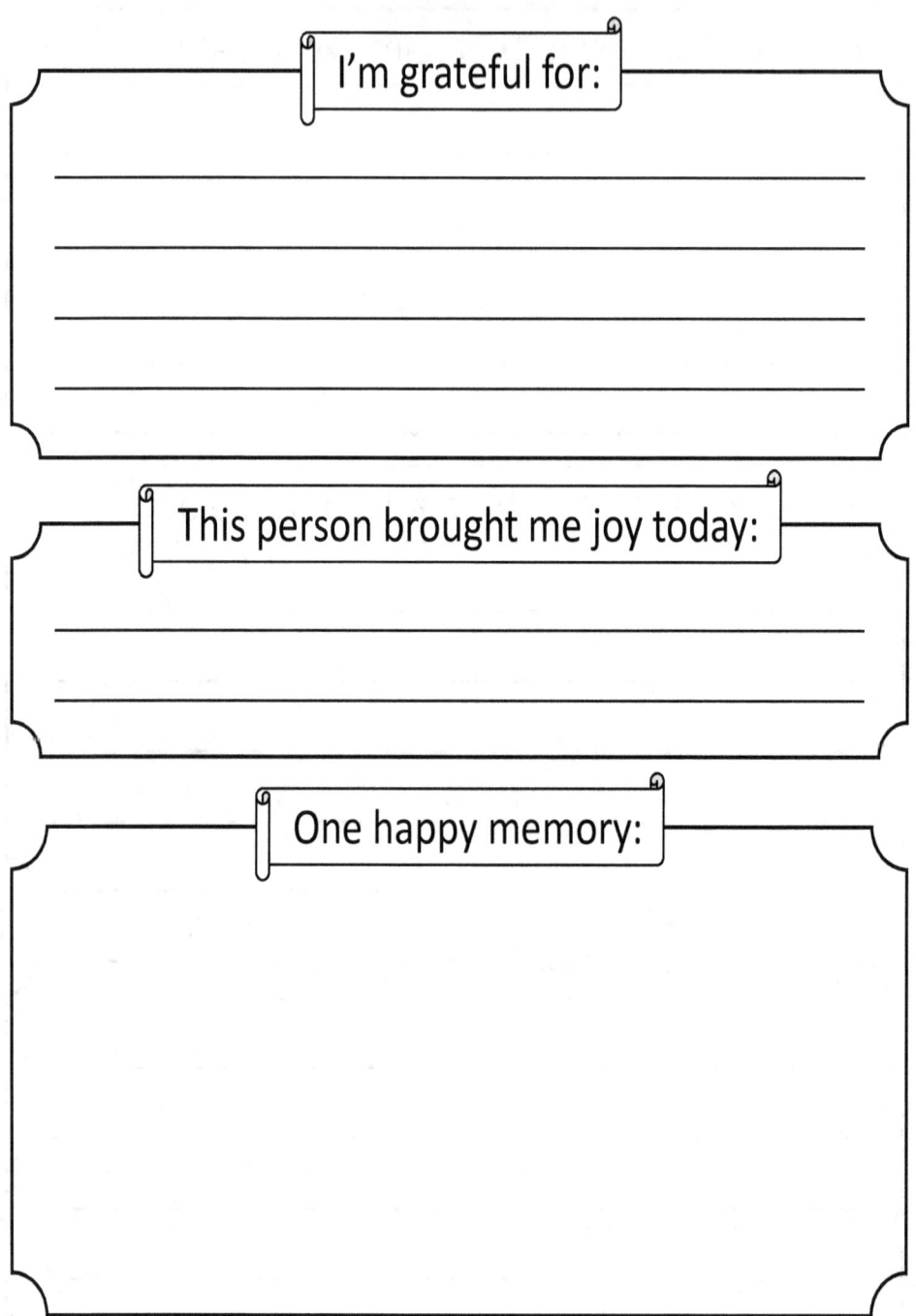

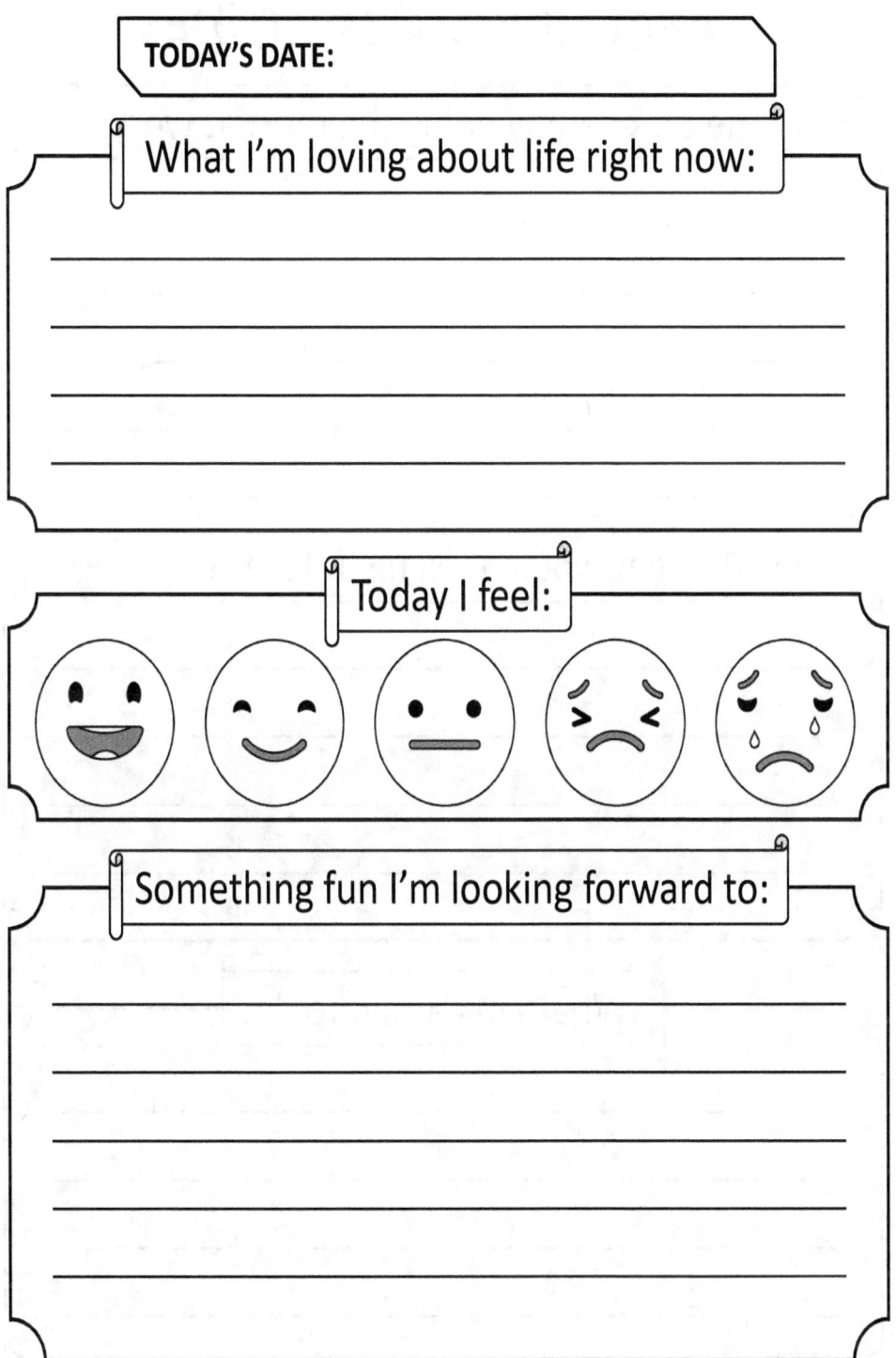

PRACTICING GRATITUDE

The task I enjoy doing the most at work:

_____
_____
_____
_____

What would I tell my future self:

_____
_____
_____
_____

What am I afraid to do:

_____
_____
_____
_____

TODAY'S DATE:

The outfit I feel the most confident in:

_____
_____
_____
_____

What would my perfect day look like:

_____
_____
_____
_____
_____

What do I need less of:

_____
_____
_____
_____

PRACTICING GRATITUDE

If I could do anything, what would it be:

_____
_____
_____
_____

Who or what inspires me the most:

_____
_____
_____
_____

What drains my energy:

_____
_____
_____
_____

TODAY'S DATE:

What is holding me back from changing:

_____
_____
_____
_____

What is something I will never forget:

_____
_____
_____
_____

What are my daily habits:

_____
_____
_____
_____

I'M GRATEFUL

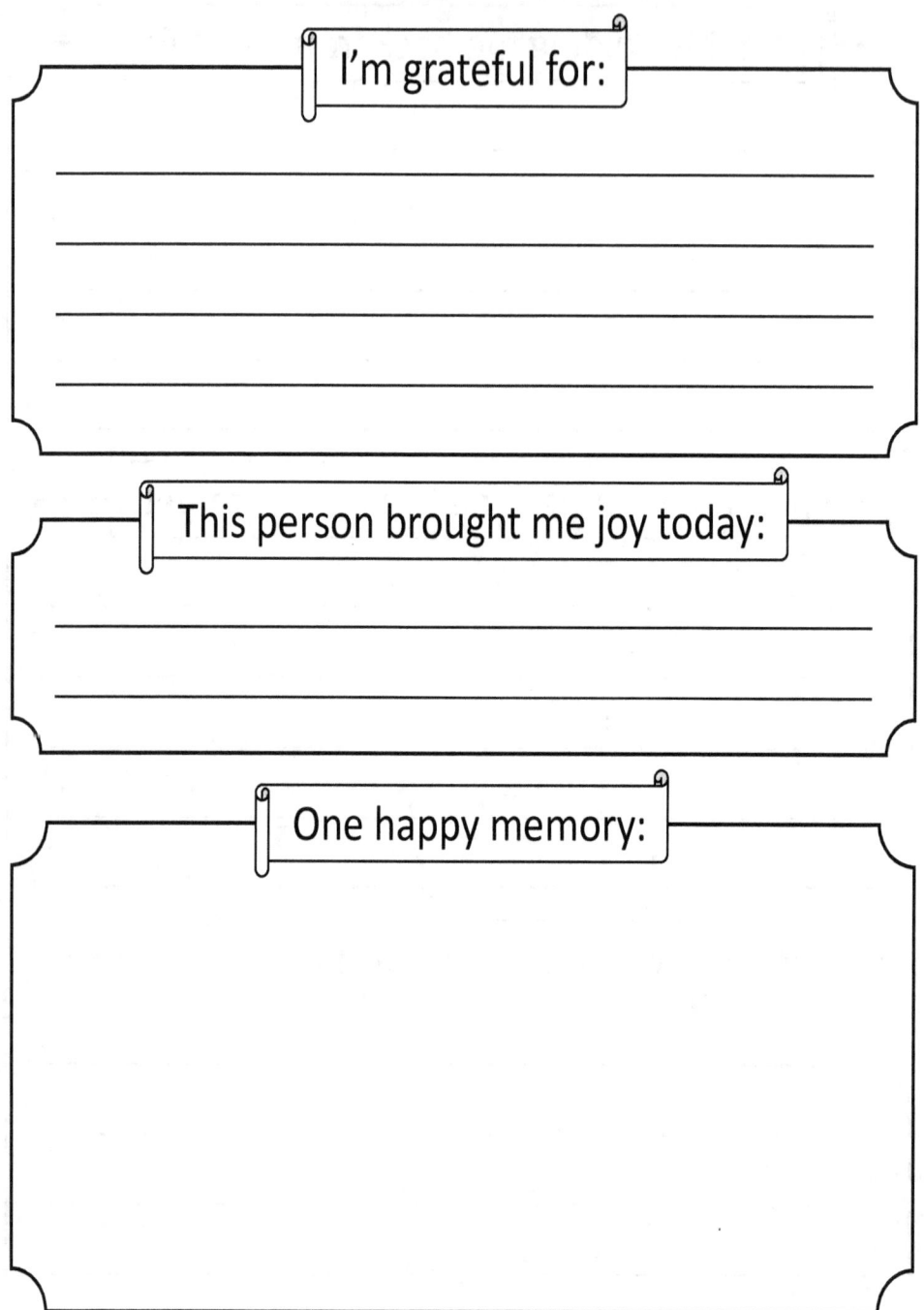

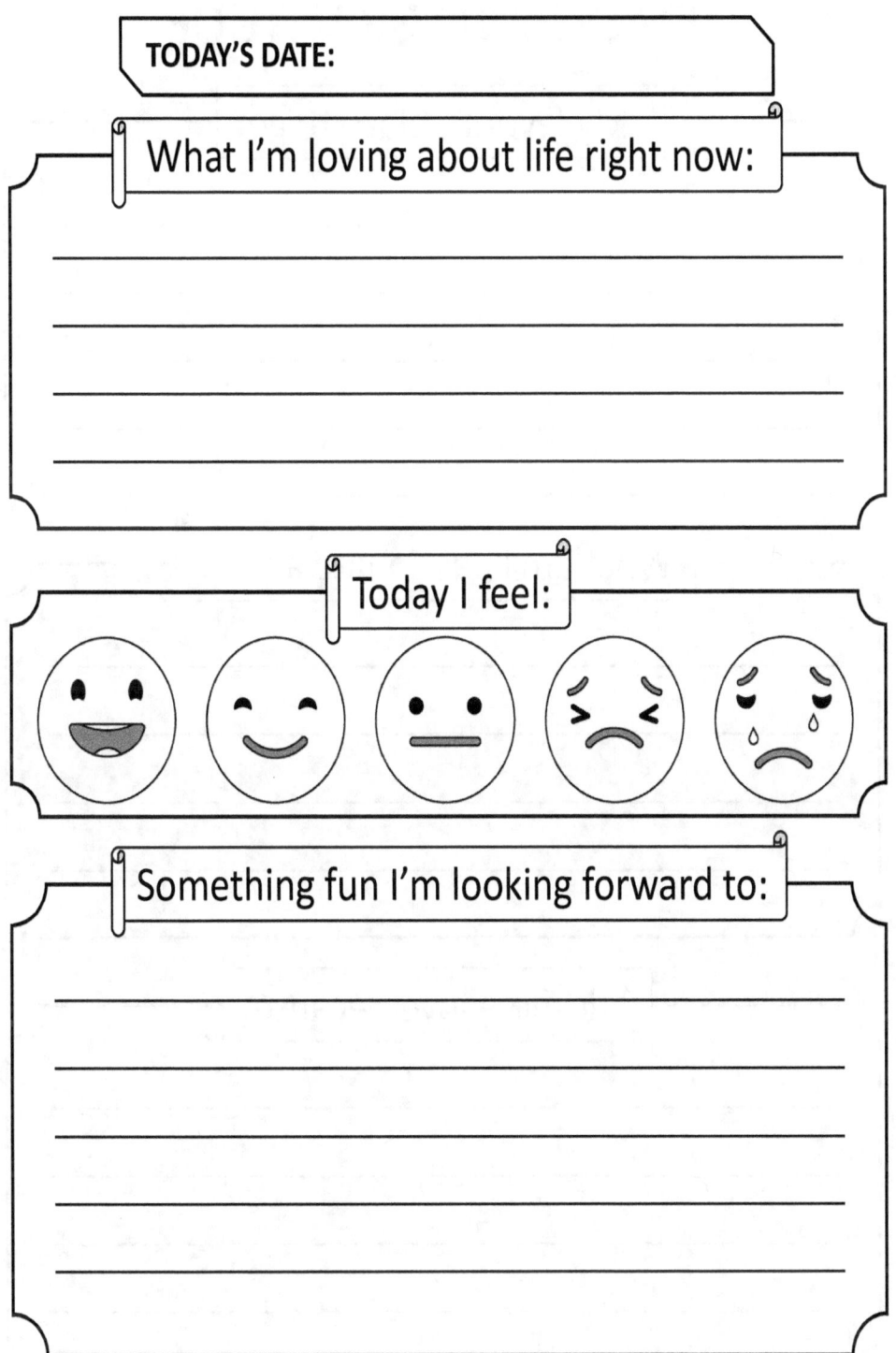

PRACTICING GRATITUDE

My favorite place to go:

_____

_____

_____

_____

What am I passionate about:

_____

_____

_____

_____

I deserve love because:

_____

_____

_____

_____

TODAY'S DATE:

Where do I want to be in the next 5 years:

___

How I do take care of myself:

___

What motivate me:

___

PRACTICING GRATITUDE

If I could travel anywhere, where would I go:

_____

_____

_____

_____

How can I love myself more:

_____

_____

_____

_____

Who makes me the happiest:

_____

_____

_____

_____

TODAY'S DATE:

What is the one piece of advice I'd give my future self:

_____
_____
_____
_____
_____

Can I improve on any of my daily habits:

_____
_____
_____
_____
_____

What makes me upset:

_____
_____
_____
_____
_____

I'M GRATEFUL

I'm grateful for:

This person brought me joy today:

One happy memory:

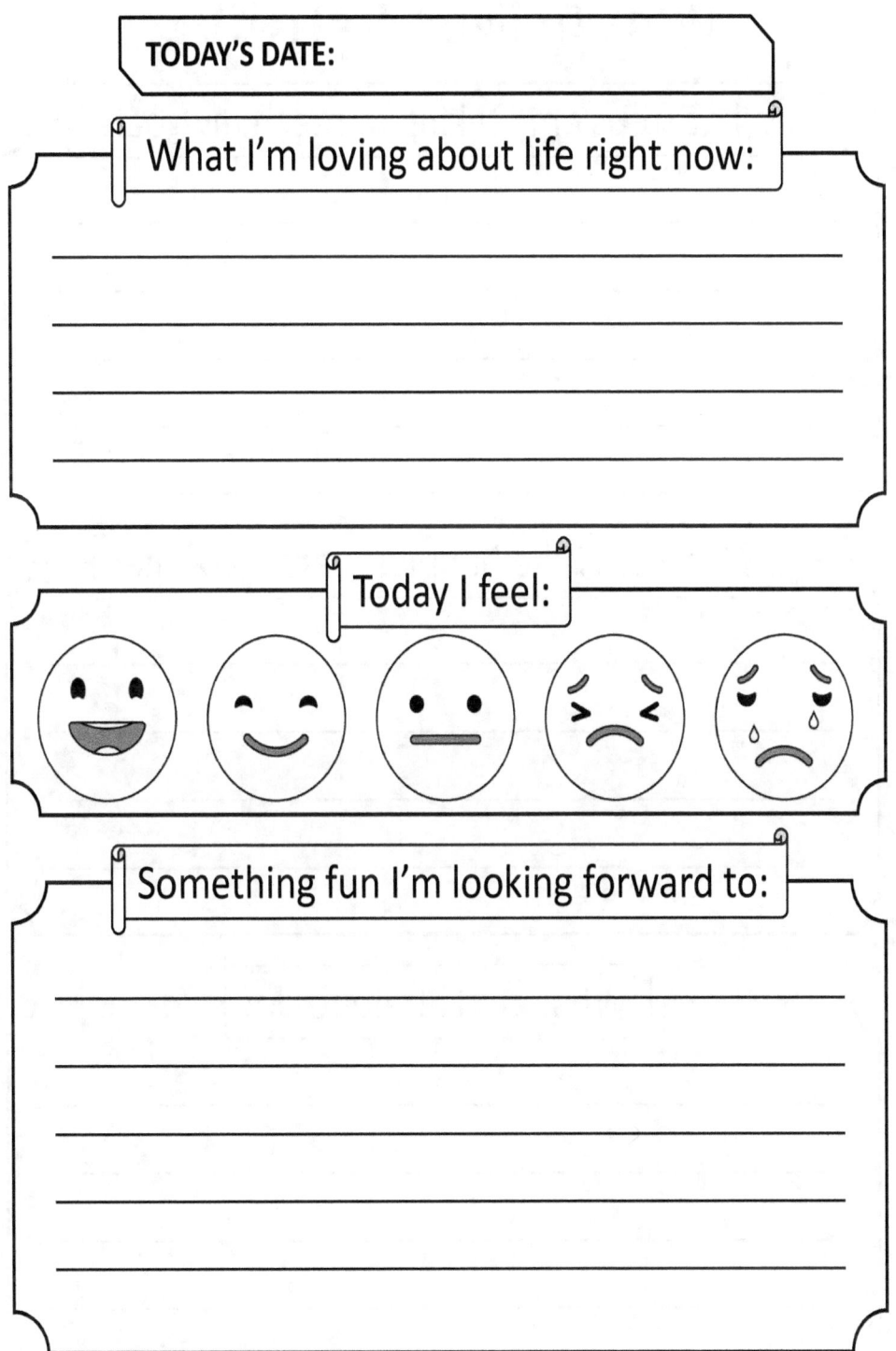

PRACTICING GRATITUDE

What steps am I taking to reach my goals:

_____
_____
_____
_____

When am I the happiest version of me:

_____
_____
_____
_____

What am I afraid to do:

_____
_____
_____
_____

TODAY'S DATE:

If I could travel anywhere, where would I go:

_____
_____
_____
_____
_____

How can I improve my daily routines:

_____
_____
_____
_____
_____

What makes me upset:

_____
_____
_____
_____
_____

I'M GRATEFUL

I'm grateful for:

_____
_____
_____
_____

This person brought me joy today:

_____
_____

One happy memory:

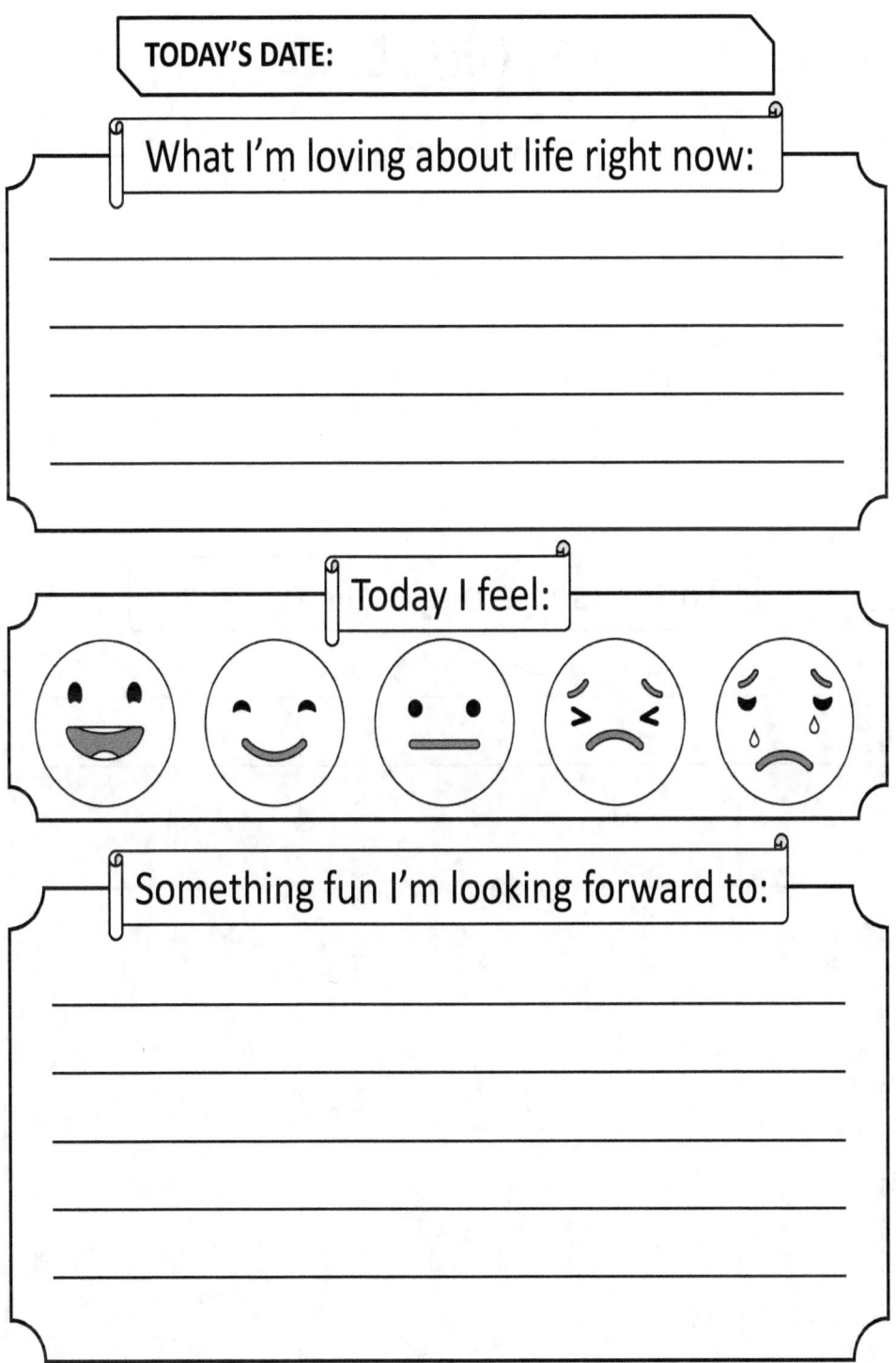

I'M GRATEFUL

I'm grateful for:

_____
_____
_____
_____

This person brought me joy today:

_____
_____

One happy memory:

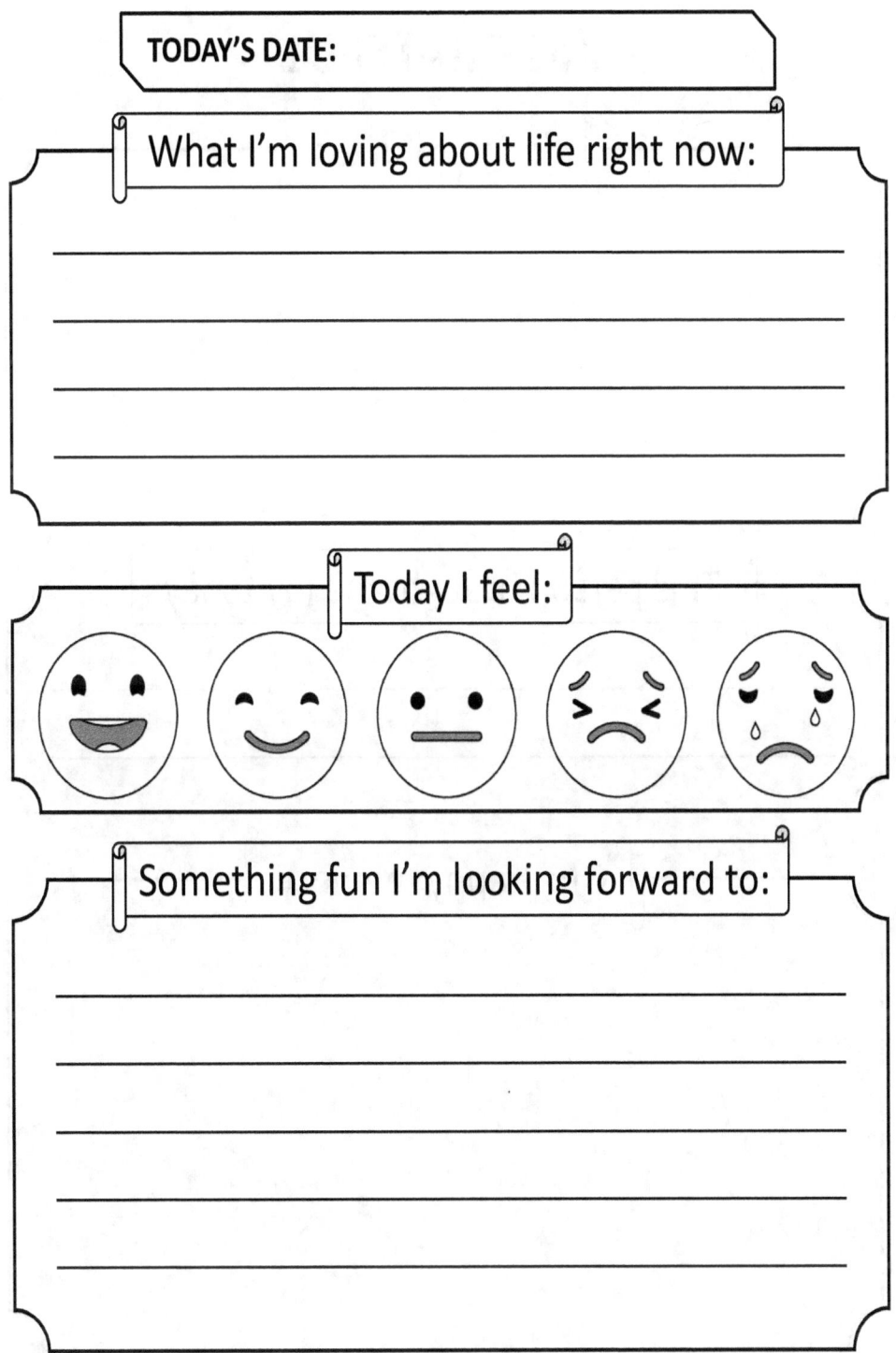

I'M GRATEFUL

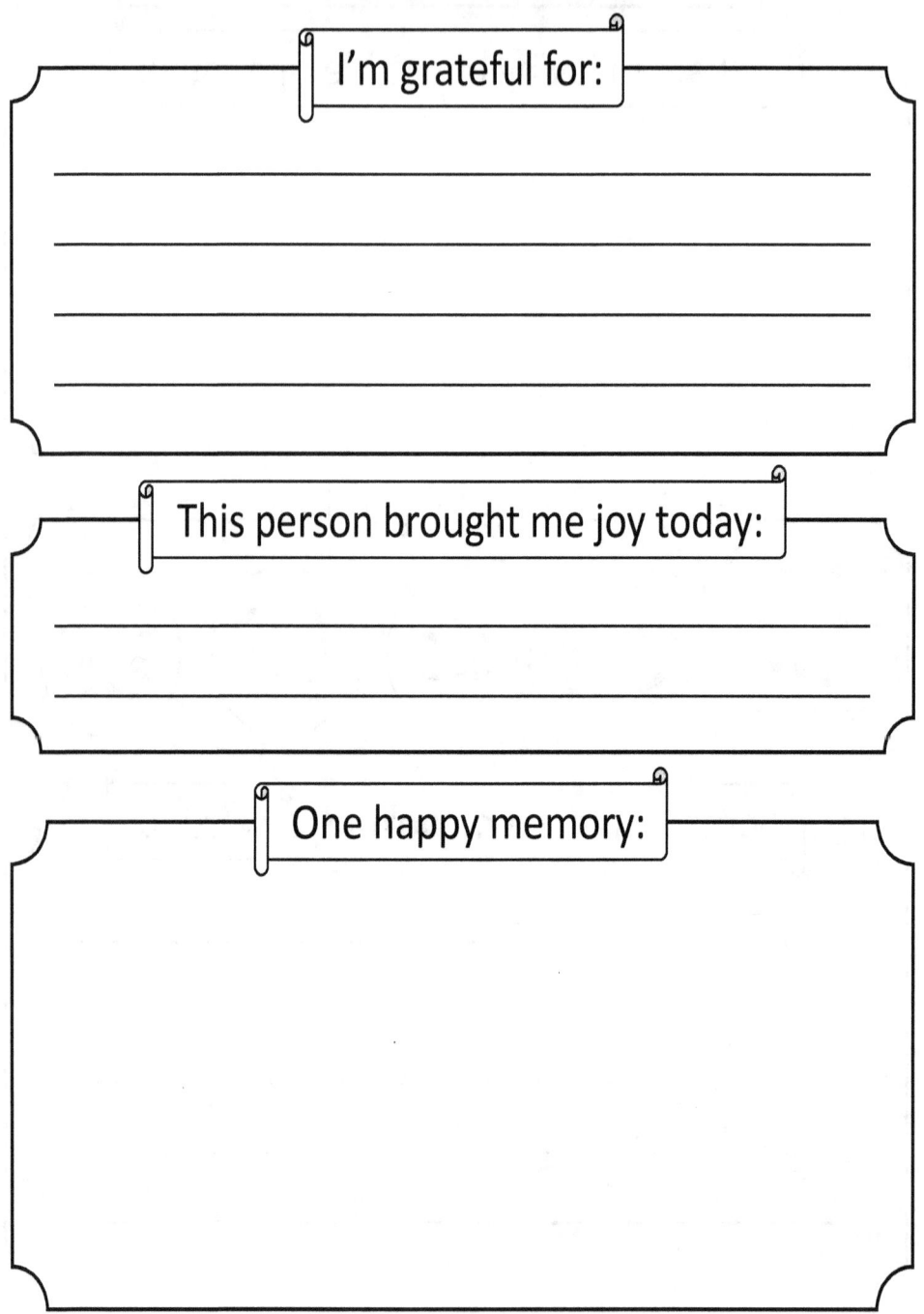

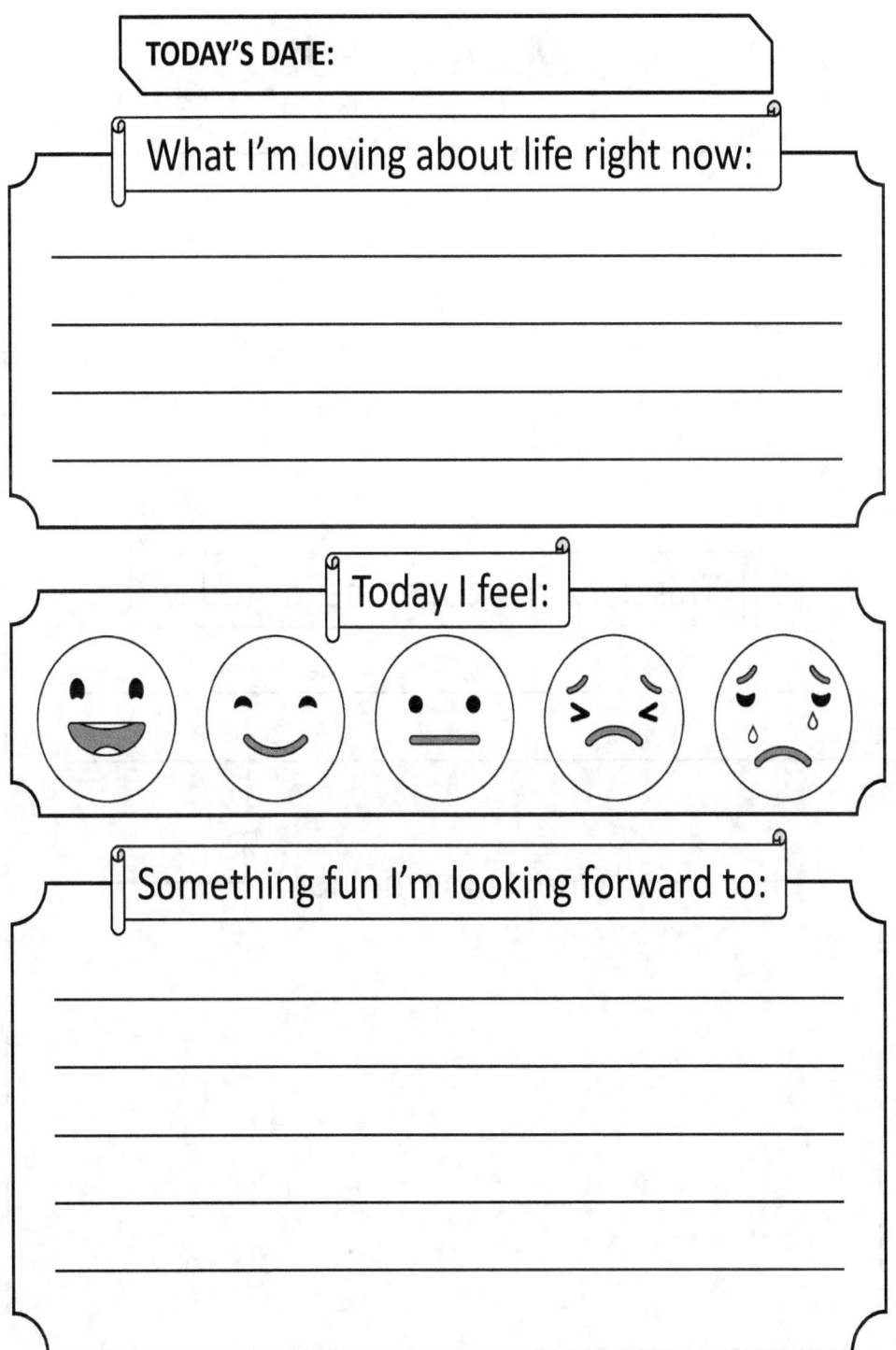

I'M GRATEFUL

I'm grateful for:

This person brought me joy today:

One happy memory:

CHANGE A HABIT IN 21 DAYS

Begin in: _____ **To:** _____

My goal is: _____

- DAY 1
- DAY 2
- DAY 3
- DAY 4
- DAY 5
- DAY 6
- DAY 7
- DAY 8
- DAY 9
- DAY 10
- DAY 11
- DAY 12
- DAY 13
- DAY 14
- DAY 15
- DAY 16
- DAY 17
- DAY 18
- DAY 19
- DAY 20
- DAY 21

How do you feel? _____

_____

_____

_____

_____

Reflect on the experience:

_____

_____

CHANGE A HABIT IN 21 DAYS

Begin in: To:

My goal is: _____

DAY 1	DAY 2	DAY 3	DAY 4	DAY 5	DAY 6
DAY 7	DAY 8	DAY 9	DAY 10	DAY 11	DAY 12
DAY 13	DAY 14	DAY 15	DAY 16	DAY 17	DAY 18
	DAY 19	DAY 20	DAY 21		

How do you feel? _____

_____

_____

_____

_____

Reflect on the experience:

_____

_____

REFRAME MY THOUGHT

SITUATION / EVENT:

Negative thought

Positive thought

ONLY POSITIVES THOUGHTS IN MY DAY

SITUATION / EVENT:

Negative thought

Positive thought

MY CONFIDENCE GOALS

What I want to achieve: _____

By: _____

Challenges: _____

_____

What I need to do:

_____

_____

_____

_____

_____

_____

_____

Result: _____

_____

Key takeaway: _____

_____

MANAGE MY FEELING

The worst feeling in my life is:
_____
_____
_____
_____

What can help me wipe away this feeling:
_____
_____
_____
_____

The best that can happen is:
_____
_____
_____

What can I do to achieve that:
_____

SHARE MORE ABOUT YOUR SELF

I'm someone who loves:

_____
_____
_____
_____

I'm someone who can:

_____
_____
_____
_____

I'm someone who has:

_____
_____
_____
_____

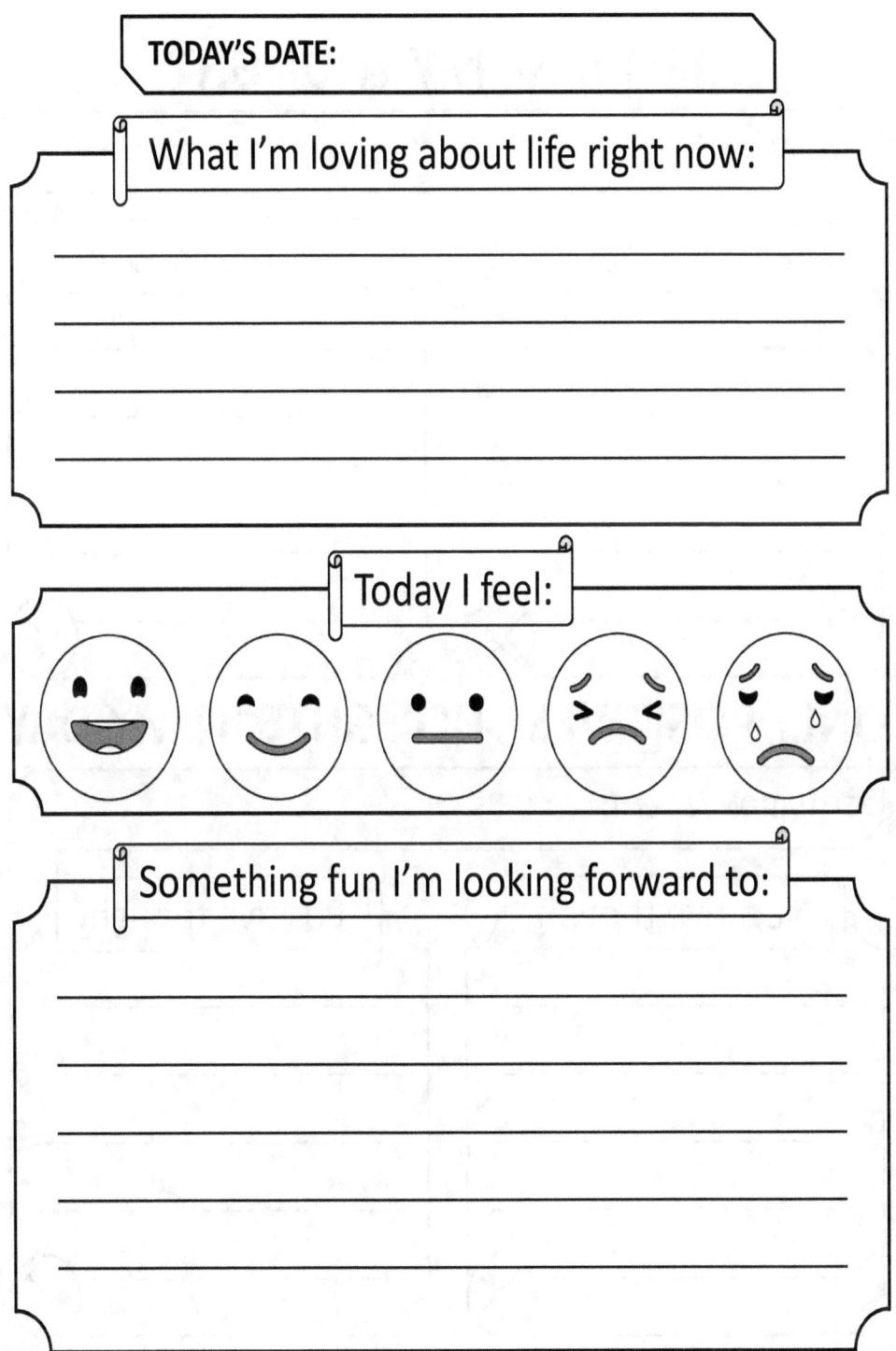

REFRAME MY THOUGHT

SITUATION / EVENT:

Negative thought

_____
_____
_____
_____
_____

Positive thought

_____
_____
_____
_____
_____

ONLY POSITIVES THOUGHTS IN MY DAY

SITUATION / EVENT:

Negative thought

_____
_____
_____
_____
_____

Positive thought

_____
_____
_____
_____
_____

TODAY'S DATE:

When I'm tired, I: _____
_____
_____
_____

When I'm stressed, I: _____
_____
_____
_____

When I'm upset, I: _____
_____
_____
_____
_____

When I'm angry, I: _____
_____
_____
_____
_____

When I feel down, I: _____
_____
_____
_____

MY CONFIDENCE GOALS

What I want to achieve: _____

By: _____

Challenges: _____

_____

What I need to do:

_____

_____

_____

_____

_____

_____

_____

Result: _____

_____

Key takeaway: _____

_____

TODAY'S DATE:

What I want to achieve: _____

By: _____

Challenges: _____

_____

What I need to do:

_____

_____

_____

_____

_____

_____

_____

_____

Result: _____

_____

Key takeaway: _____

_____

I'M GRATEFUL

I'm grateful for:

This person brought me joy today:

One happy memory:

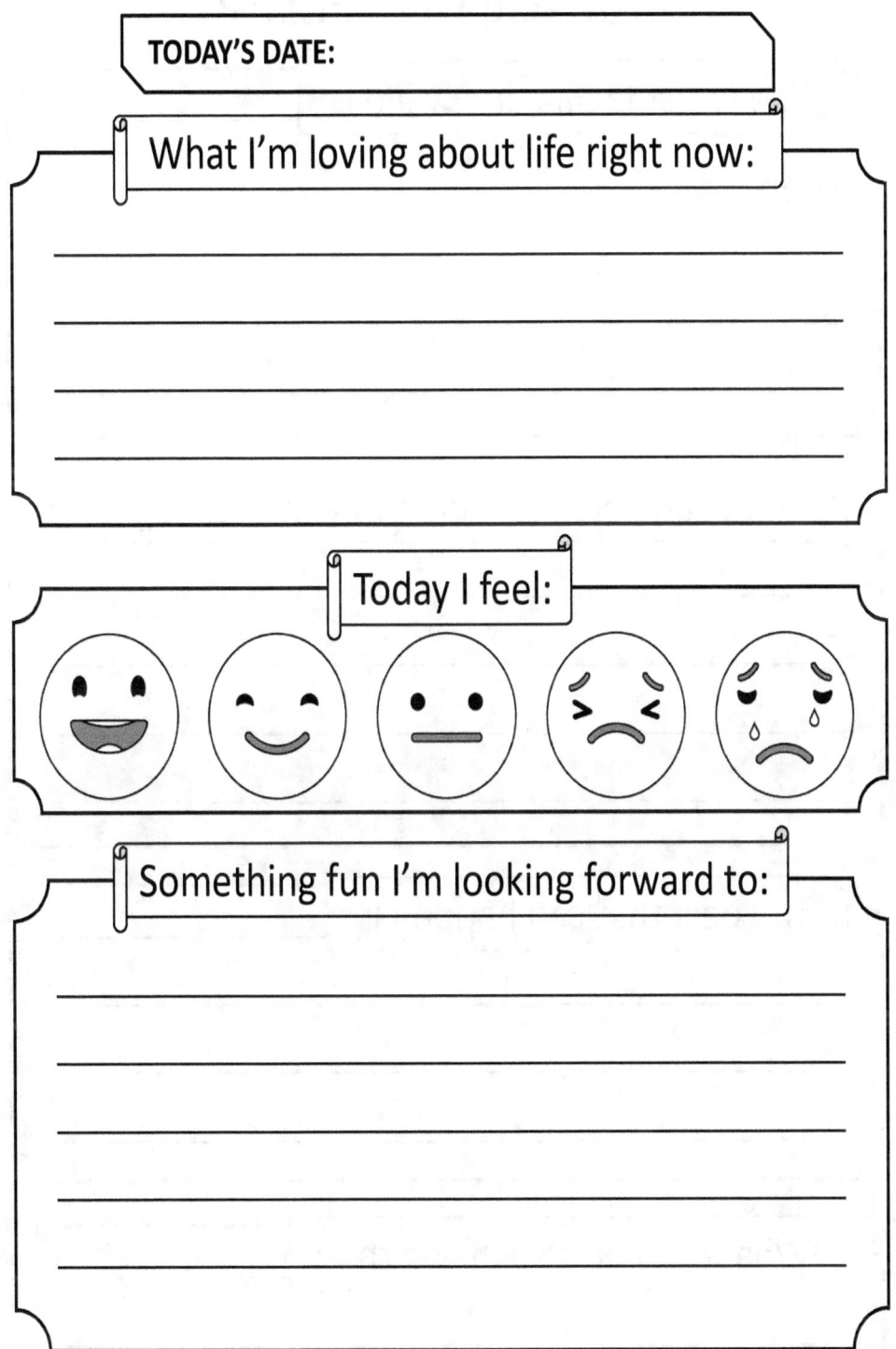

MANAGE MY FEELING

The worst feeling in my life is:
_____
_____
_____
_____

What can help me wipe away this feeling:
_____
_____
_____
_____

The best that can happen is:
_____
_____
_____

What can I do to achieve that:
_____
_____

TODAY'S DATE:

The best feeling in my life is:

Say something nice about you/your life:

I'M GRATEFUL

I'm grateful for:

This person brought me joy today:

One happy memory:

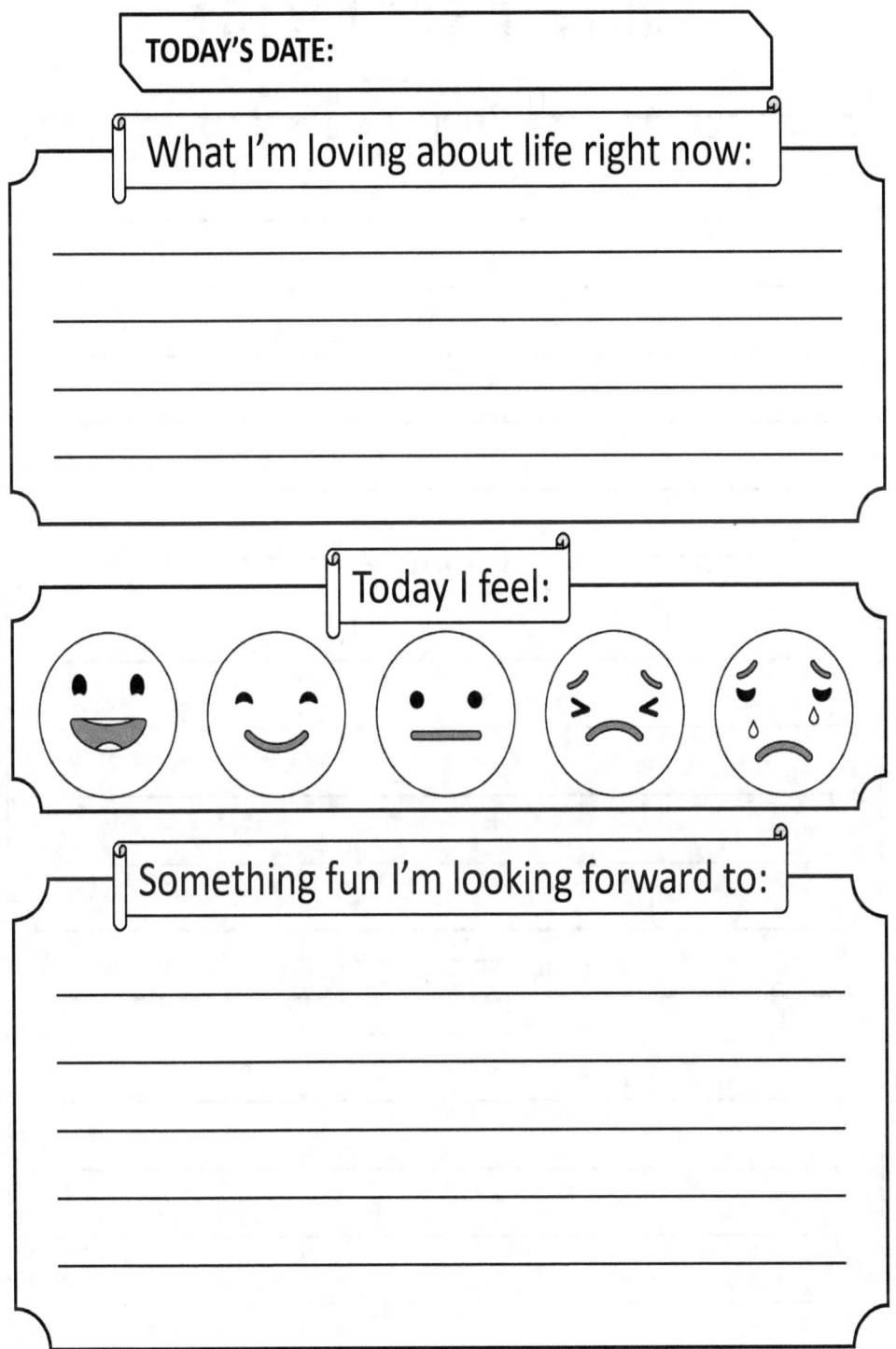

PRIORITIES OF MY LIFE

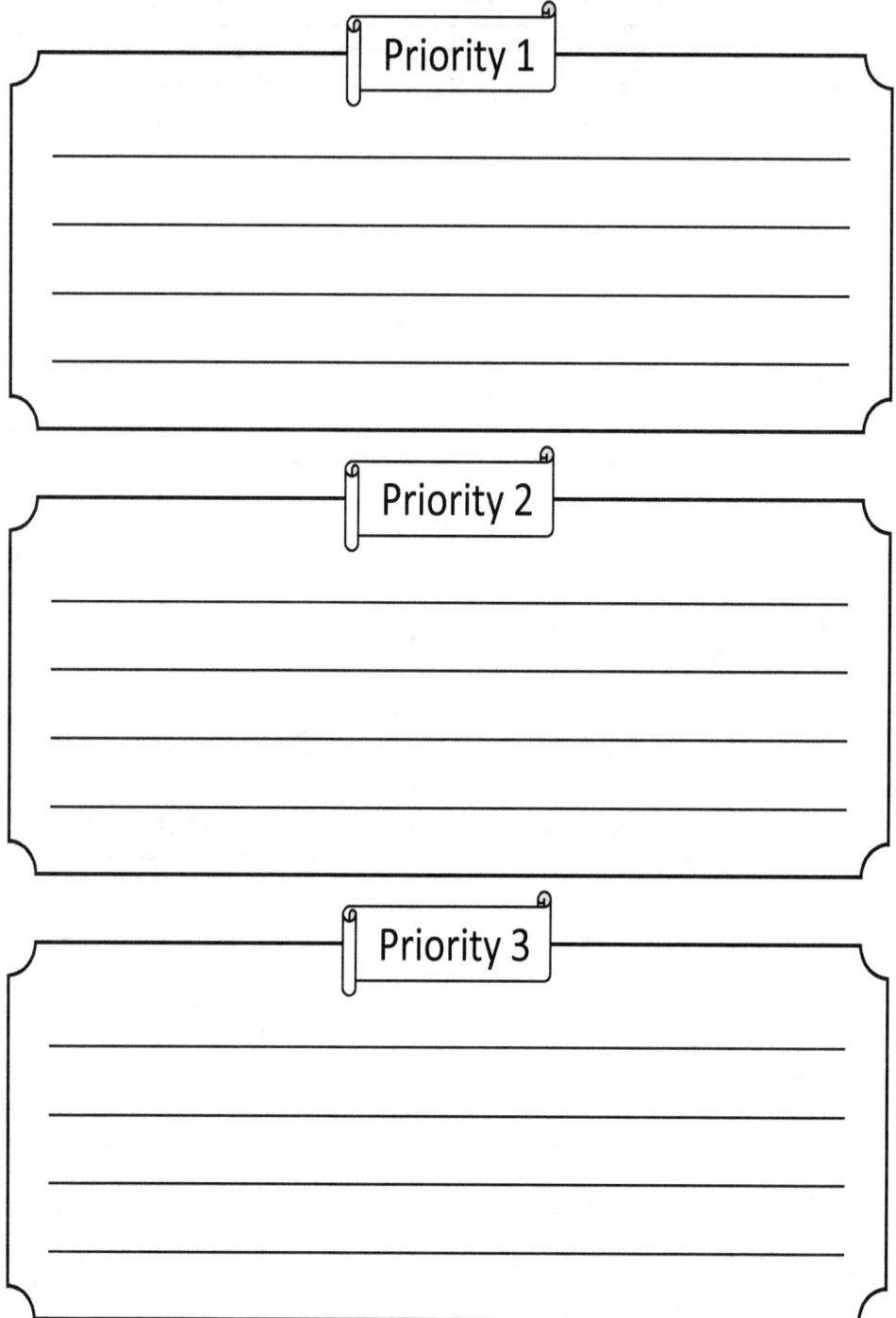

TODAY'S DATE:

Priority 4

Priority 5

Priority 6

SHARE MORE ABOUT YOUR SELF

I'm someone who loves:

_____
_____
_____
_____

I'm someone who can:

_____
_____
_____
_____

I'm someone who has:

_____
_____
_____
_____

TODAY'S DATE:

I'm someone who wishes:

I'm someone who is thankful for:

I'm someone who never forgets to:

I'M GRATEFUL

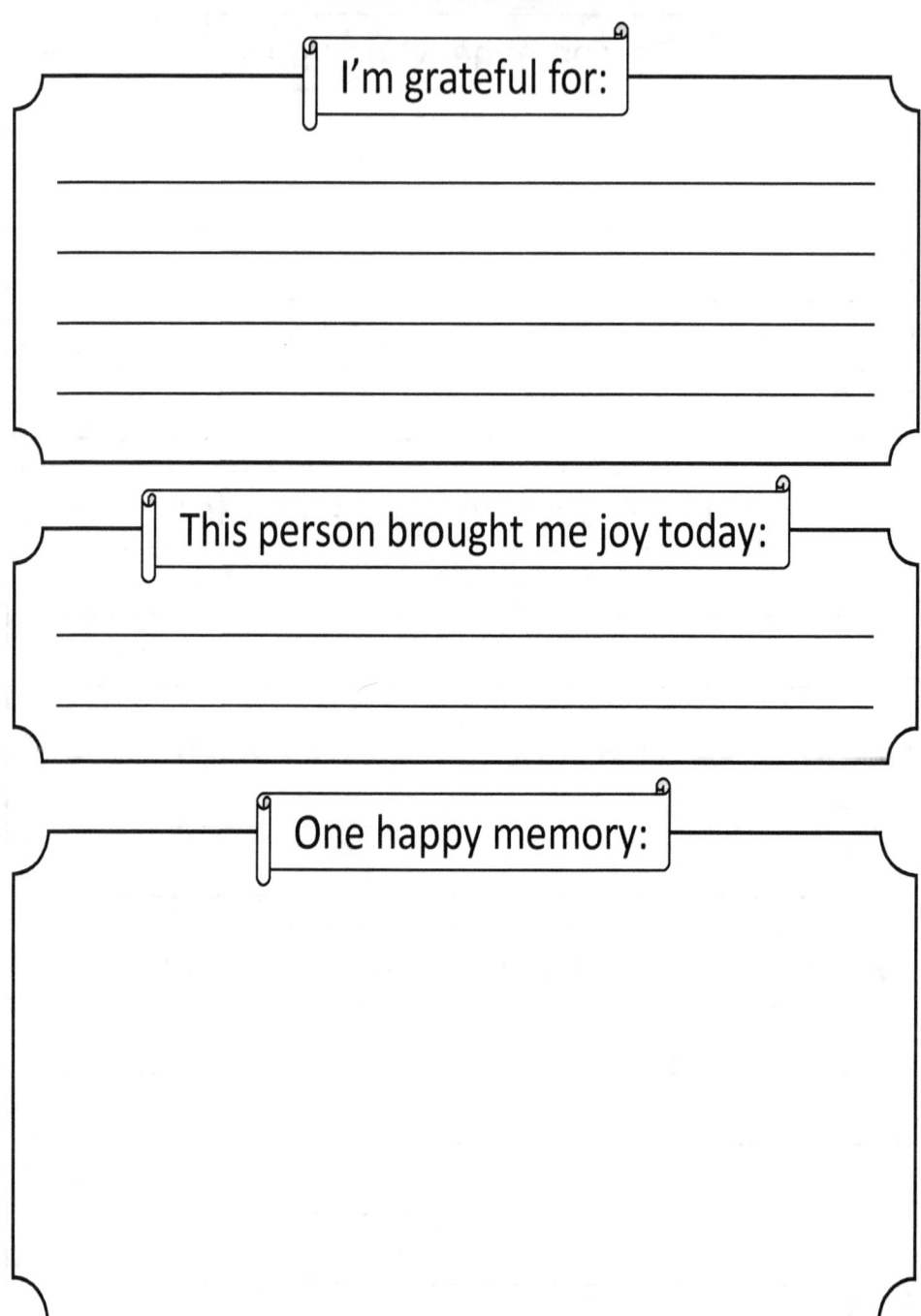

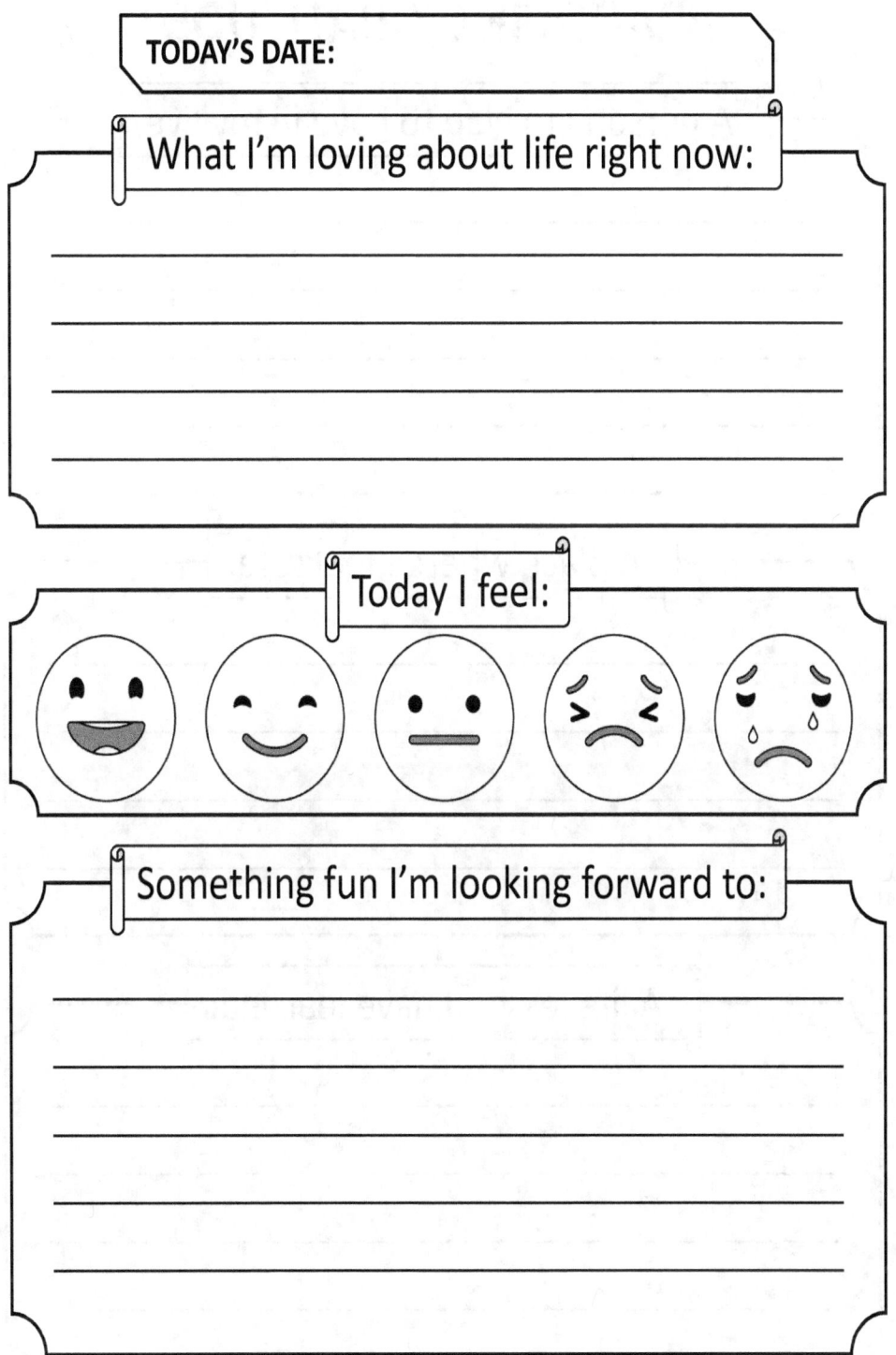

PRACTICING GRATITUDE

A person I'm glad to have in my live:

A place where I feel safe:

A life lesson I have learned:

TODAY'S DATE:

A characteristic of my home that I love:

_____
_____
_____
_____

My favorite aspect of my personality:

_____
_____
_____
_____

A book that I loved reading:

_____
_____
_____
_____

PRACTICING GRATITUDE

My favorite song that improves my mind:

_____
_____
_____
_____

A memory that makes me smile:

_____
_____
_____
_____

My favorite food or meal:

_____
_____
_____
_____

TODAY'S DATE:

A future event that I am excited about:

An accomplishment I am proud of:

My favorite time of the day:

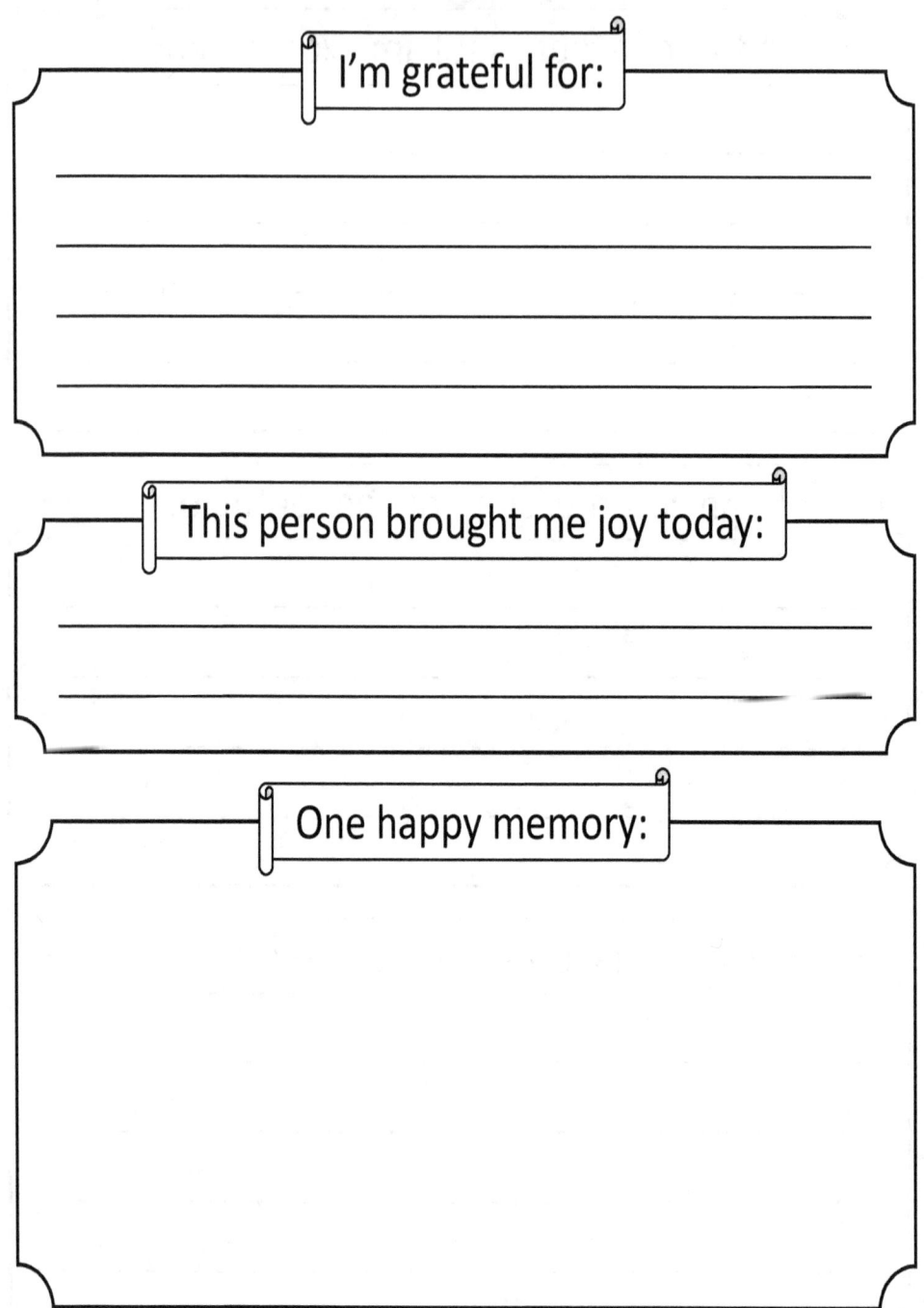

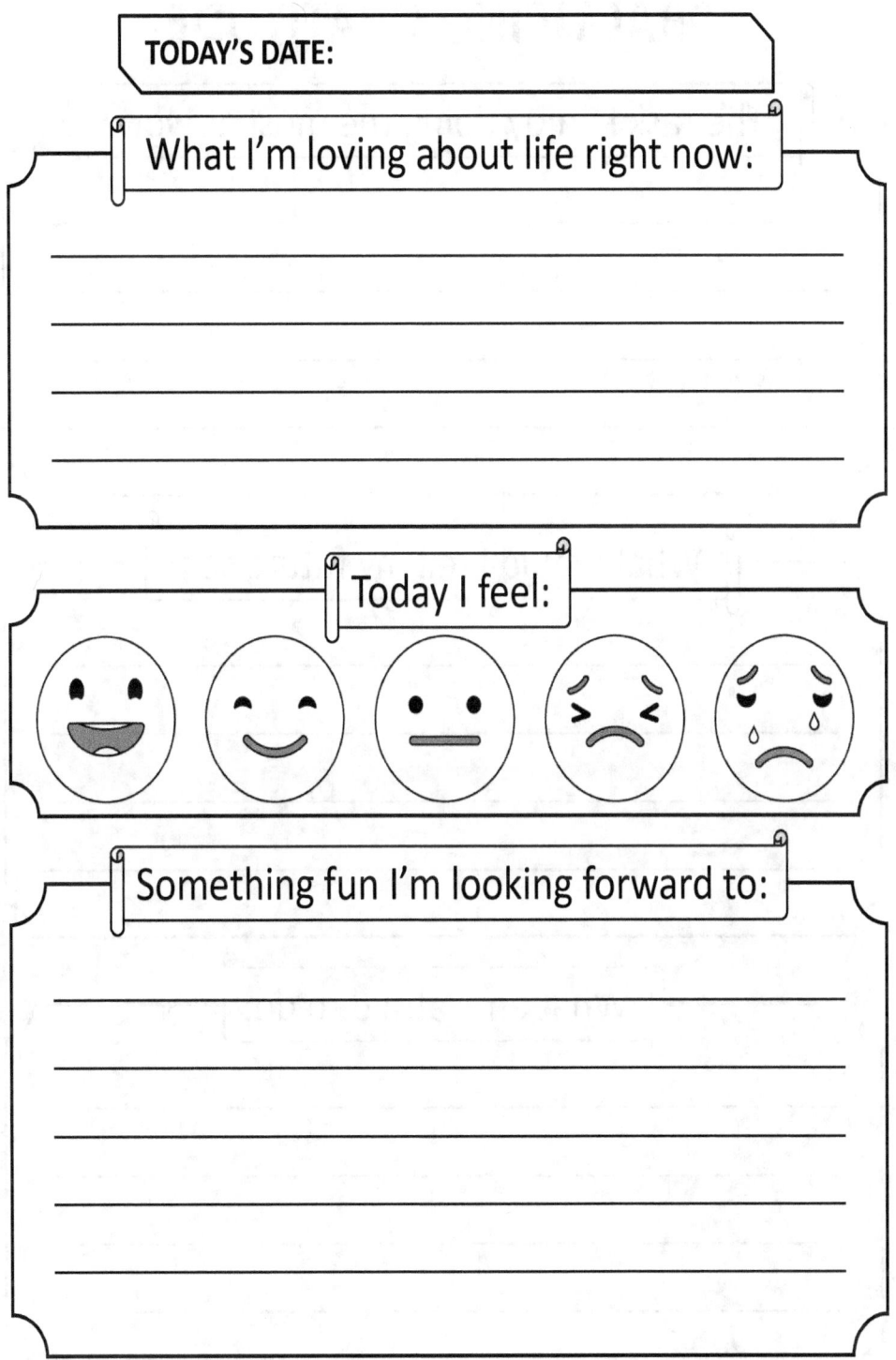

PRACTICING GRATITUDE

The task I enjoy doing the most at work:

_____
_____
_____
_____

What would I tell my future self:

_____
_____
_____
_____

What am I afraid to do:

_____
_____
_____
_____

TODAY'S DATE:

The outfit I feel the most confident in:
_____
_____
_____
_____

What would my perfect day look like:
_____
_____
_____
_____

What do I need less of:
_____
_____
_____
_____

PRACTICING GRATITUDE

If I could do anything, what would it be:

_____
_____
_____
_____

Who or what inspires me the most:

_____
_____
_____
_____

What drains my energy:

_____
_____
_____
_____

TODAY'S DATE:

What is holding me back from changing:
_____
_____
_____
_____

What is something I will never forget:
_____
_____
_____
_____

What are my daily habits:
_____
_____
_____
_____

I'M GRATEFUL

I'm grateful for:

_____

_____

_____

_____

This person brought me joy today:

_____

_____

One happy memory:

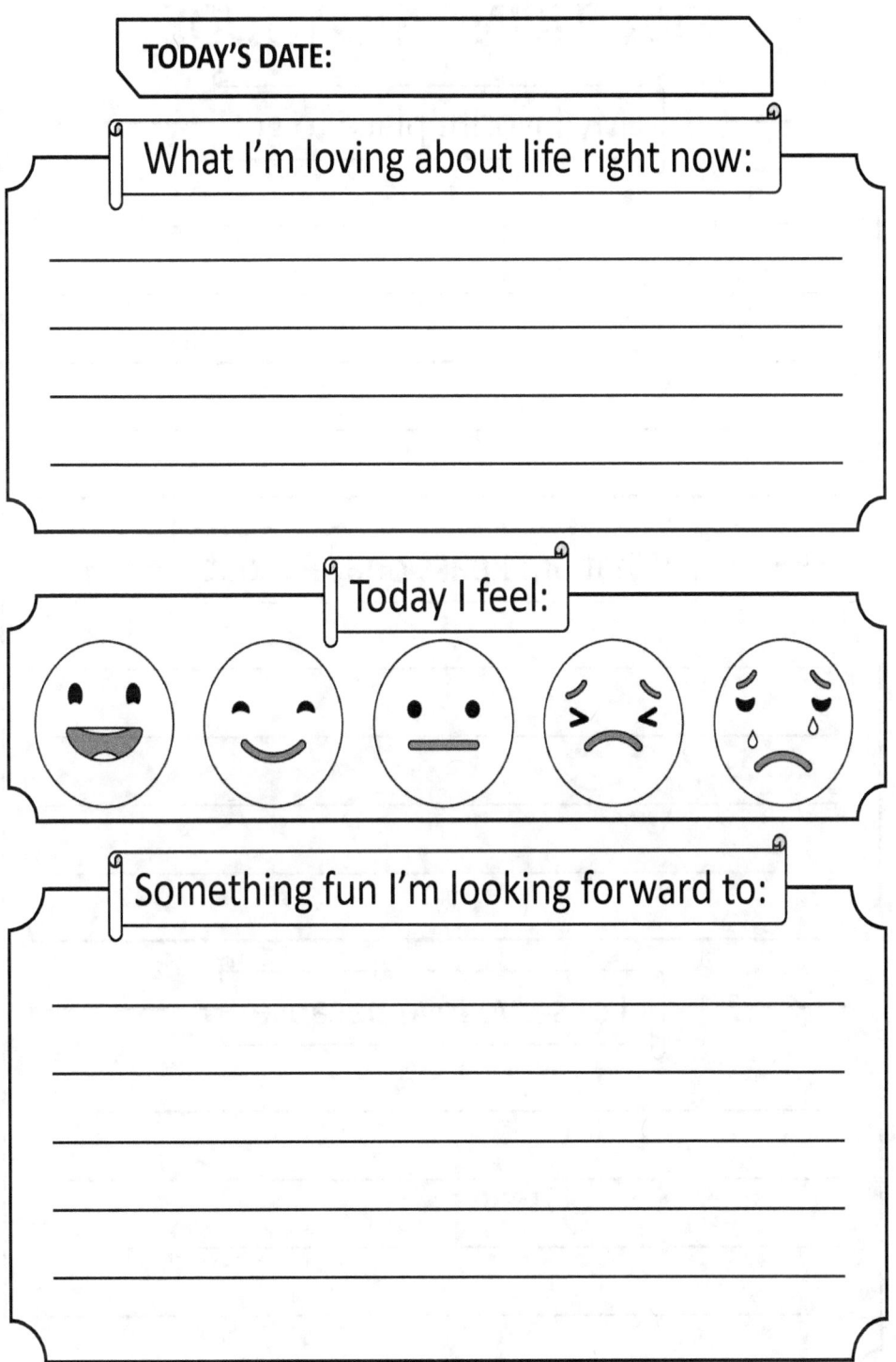

TODAY'S DATE:

What I'm loving about life right now:

Today I feel:

Something fun I'm looking forward to:

PRACTICING GRATITUDE

My favorite place to go:

_____

_____

_____

_____

What am I passionate about:

_____

_____

_____

_____

I deserve love because:

_____

_____

_____

_____

TODAY'S DATE:

Where do I want to be in the next 5 years:
_____
_____
_____
_____

How I do take care of myself:
_____
_____
_____
_____

What motivate me:
_____
_____
_____
_____

PRACTICING GRATITUDE

If I could travel anywhere, where would I go:

_____
_____
_____
_____

How can I love myself more:

_____
_____
_____
_____

Who makes me the happiest:

_____
_____
_____
_____

TODAY'S DATE:

What is the one piece of advice I'd give my future self:
_____
_____
_____
_____

Can I improve on any of my daily habits:
_____
_____
_____
_____

What makes me upset:
_____
_____
_____
_____

I'M GRATEFUL

I'm grateful for:

_____

_____

_____

_____

This person brought me joy today:

_____

_____

One happy memory:

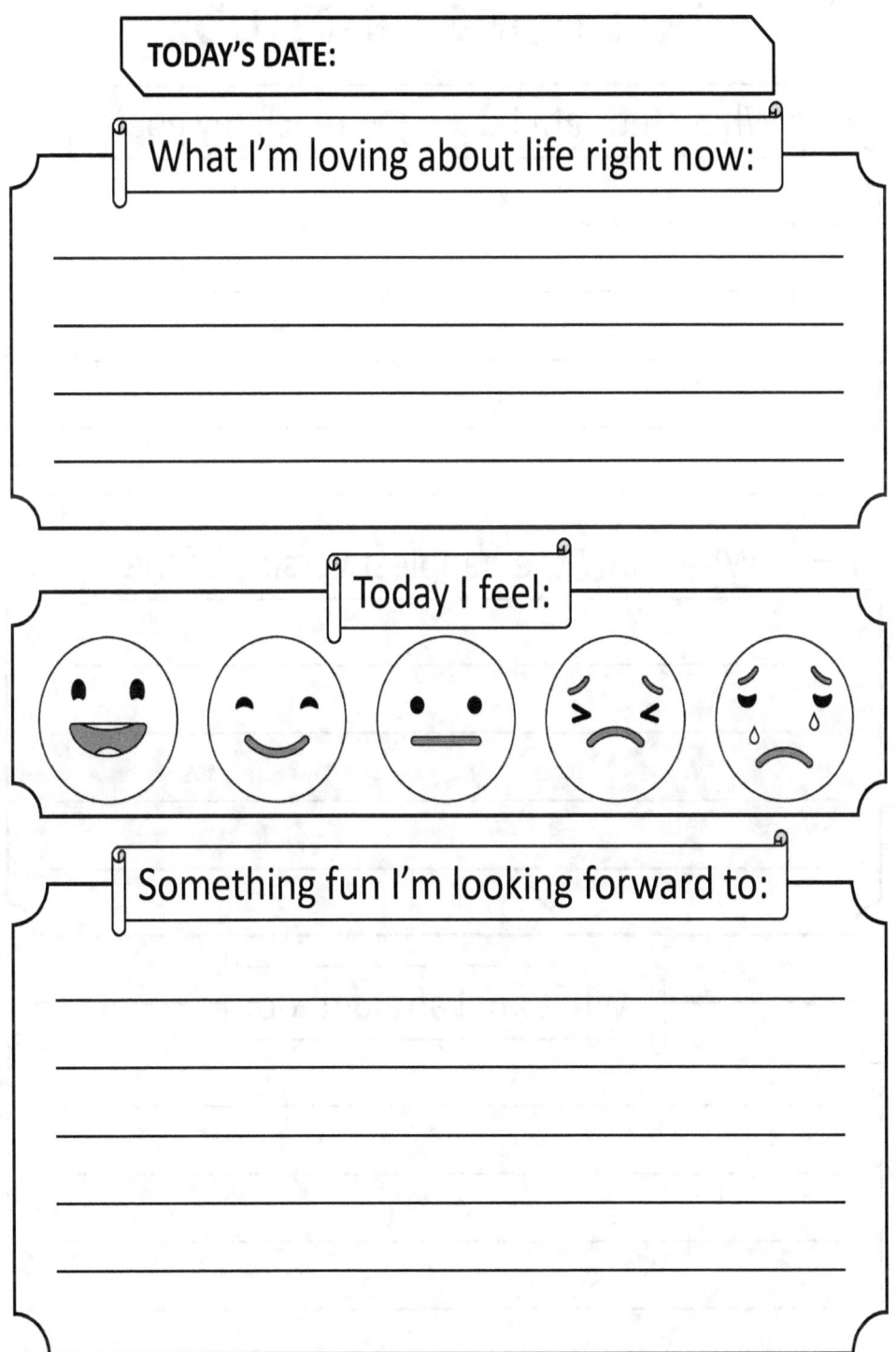

PRACTICING GRATITUDE

What steps am I taking to reach my goals:

_____
_____
_____

When am I the happiest version of me:

_____
_____
_____

What am I afraid to do:

_____
_____
_____

TODAY'S DATE:

If I could travel anywhere, where would I go:

_____
_____
_____
_____
_____

How can I improve my daily routines:

_____
_____
_____
_____
_____

What makes me upset:

_____
_____
_____
_____
_____

I'M GRATEFUL

I'm grateful for:

This person brought me joy today:

One happy memory:

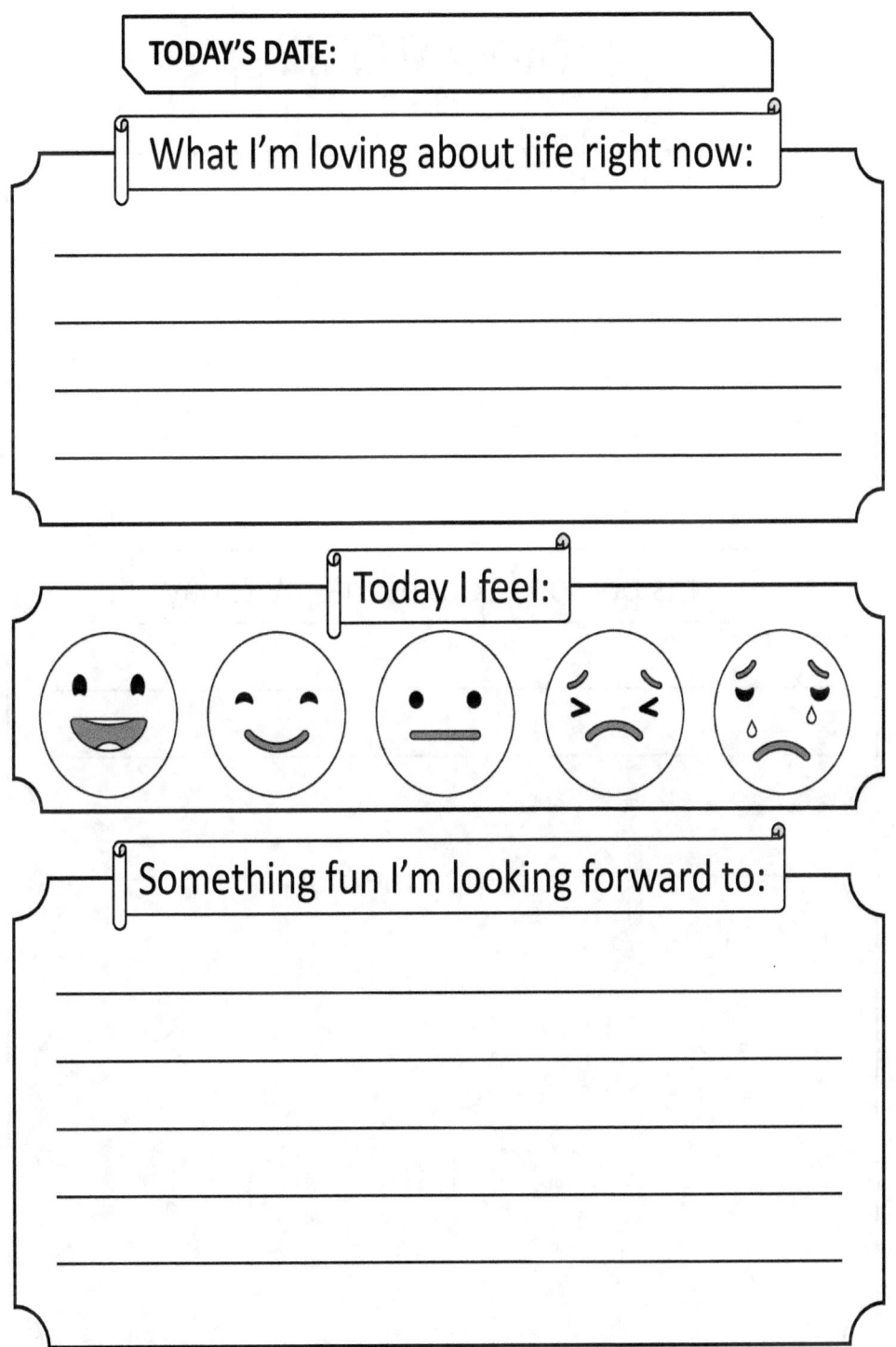

I'M GRATEFUL

I'm grateful for:

This person brought me joy today:

One happy memory:

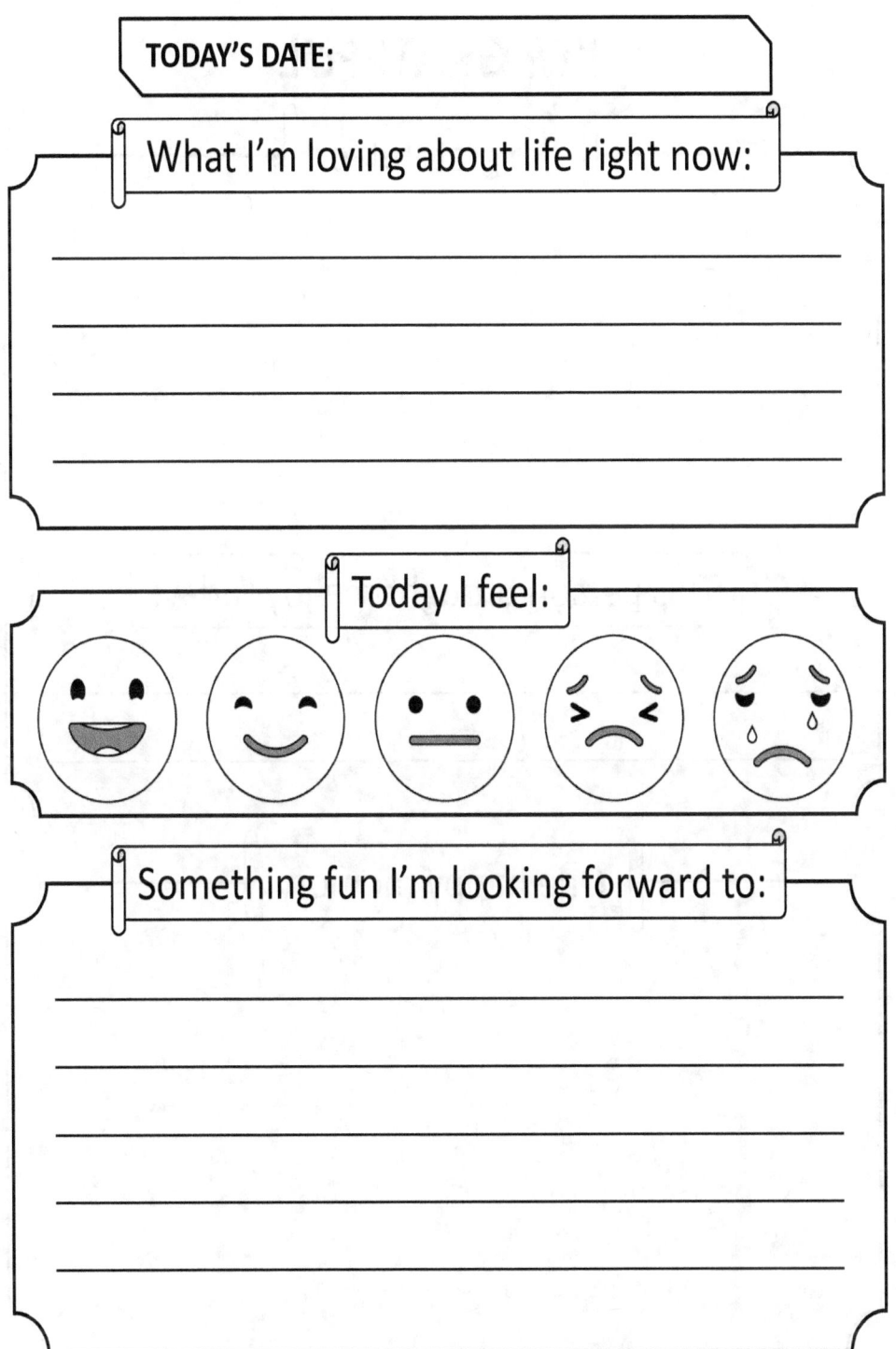

I'M GRATEFUL

I'm grateful for:

This person brought me joy today:

One happy memory:

TODAY'S DATE:

What I'm loving about life right now:

_____
_____
_____
_____

Today I feel:

Something fun I'm looking forward to:

_____
_____
_____
_____
_____

I'M GRATEFUL

I'm grateful for:

_____

_____

_____

_____

This person brought me joy today:

_____

_____

One happy memory:

CHANGE A HABIT IN 21 DAYS

Begin in: _____ To: _____

My goal is: _____

< DAY 1 > < DAY 2 > < DAY 3 > < DAY 4 > < DAY 5 > < DAY 6 >
< DAY 7 > < DAY 8 > < DAY 9 > < DAY 10 > < DAY 11 > < DAY 12 >
< DAY 13 > < DAY 14 > < DAY 15 > < DAY 16 > < DAY 17 > < DAY 18 >
< DAY 19 > < DAY 20 > < DAY 21 >

How do you feel? _____

_____

_____

_____

_____

Reflect on the experience:

_____

_____

CHANGE A HABIT IN 21 DAYS

Begin in: _____ **To:** _____

My goal is: _____

DAY 1	DAY 2	DAY 3	DAY 4	DAY 5	DAY 6
DAY 7	DAY 8	DAY 9	DAY 10	DAY 11	DAY 12
DAY 13	DAY 14	DAY 15	DAY 16	DAY 17	DAY 18
		DAY 19	DAY 20	DAY 21	

How do you feel? _____

_____

_____

_____

_____

Reflect on the experience:

_____

_____

Hey there!!!

We hope you enjoyed our book. As a small family company, your feedback is very important to us. Please let us know how you like our book at:
believepublisher@gmail.com

Without your voice we don't exist!

Please, support us and leave a review!

Thank you!!!

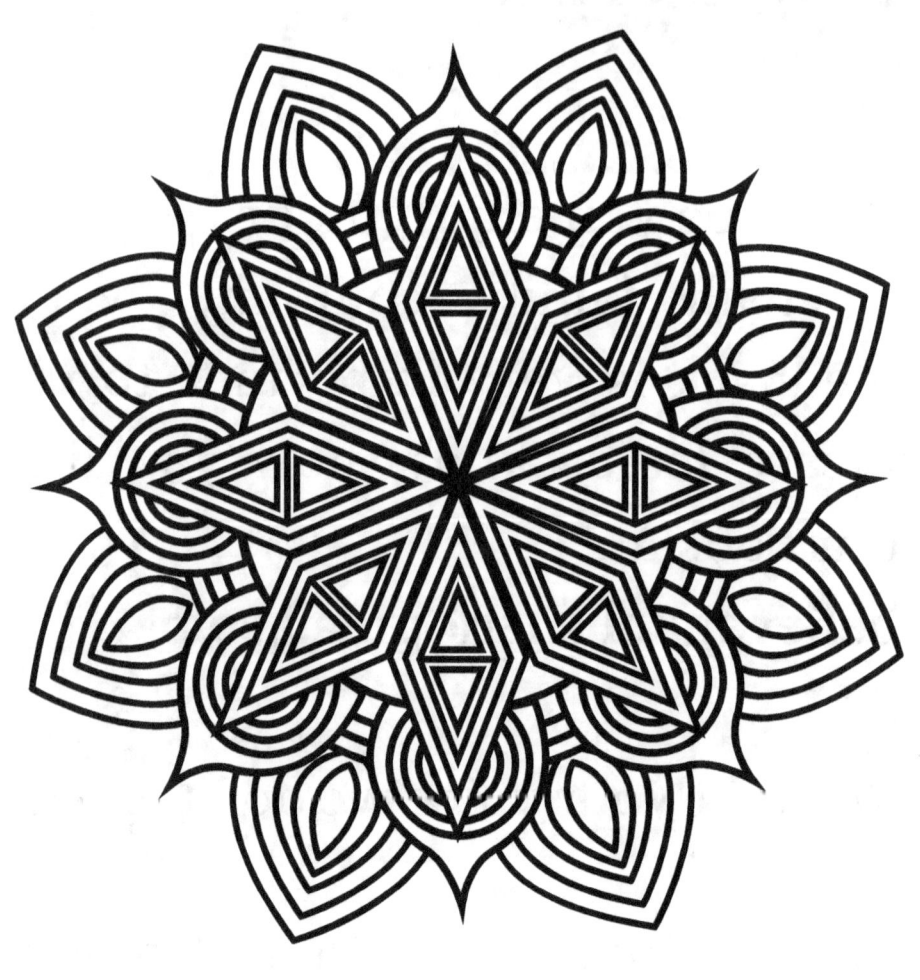

www.ingramcontent.com/pod-product-compliance
Lightning Source LLC
LaVergne TN
LVHW020424080526
838202LV00055B/5025